The Cancer Solution
Taking Charge of Your Life with Cancer

*A Cancer Handbook for Inquisitive
Laypersons and Health Care Professionals*

Jack C. Westman, M.D., M.S.

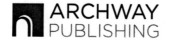

ARCHWAY
PUBLISHING

Archway Publishing books may be ordered through booksellers or by contacting:

Archway Publishing
1663 Liberty Drive
Bloomington, IN 47403
www.archwaypublishing.com
1-(888)-242-5904

Because of the dynamic nature of the Internet, any web addresses or links contained in this book may have changed since publication and may no longer be valid. The views expressed in this work are solely those of the author and do not necessarily reflect the views of the publisher, and the publisher hereby disclaims any responsibility for them.

Any people depicted in stock imagery provided by Thinkstock are models, and such images are being used for illustrative purposes only.
Certain stock imagery © Thinkstock.

ISBN: 978-1-4808-1308-3 (sc)
ISBN: 978-1-4808-1310-6 (hc)
ISBN: 978-1-4808-1309-0 (e)

Library of Congress Control Number: 2014922399

Printed in the United States of America.

Archway Publishing rev. date: 1/28/2015

The information, ideas, and suggestions in this book are not intended as a substitute for professional medical advice. Before following any suggestions contained in this book, you should consult your personal physician. Neither the author nor the publisher shall be liable or responsible for any loss or damage allegedly arising as a consequence of your use or application of any information or suggestions in this book.

There will be a major change in the way cancer is treated over the next ten years. If you or a loved one is receiving cancer care, you can take charge of your cancer treatment now by complementing it through diet and nutritional supplements that have been shown to prevent cancer and reverse its growth and by having knowledge about your cancer that you can share with your doctors.

Dedicated to

Conrad Alexander Westman
Linda Lee Swanson Branch
Nancy Kathryn Baehre Westman

Contents

Preface

My beloved wife Nancy's 34 years of life with cancer and ultimate debilitating process of dying from cancer in 2012 compelled me to learn all that I could about cancer research and treatment. The appearance of cancer in two relatives and the urging of friends clinched my determination to share what I have learned with persons affected by cancer and with other health care professionals.

Cancer inevitably will affect your life directly or through those close to you as it has mine. This may be why you are reading this book and seeking a perspective on the world's most devastating disease that will be the cause of death for one of three of us in the United States. I have written this book to be readable for lay persons and yet contain useful technical details for health care professionals. This book essentially is a handbook to be skimmed at first reading and used for later reference as needed.

A growing body of evidence shows that patients who are inquisitive about and actively involved in their health care have better health outcomes and incur lower costs. As a result, many public and private health care organizations are educating people about their conditions and involving them more fully in making decisions about their care. I am following this trend.

I wish that I could be writing about how we are winning the War on Cancer. Unfortunately, I must join the ranks of objective observers of the current state of cancer research and care and acknowledge that we are far short of winning that War.

I wrote this book for you with four aims. The first is to give you a broad overview of the different forms of cancer treatment and cancer research in as understandable terms as I can. The second is to provide enough technical details so that you can use this book as a reference for questions about specific aspects of cancer. The third is to stimulate your interest in complementary cancer care. The fourth is to encourage you as a layperson or a professional to become an informed advocate for federal and private funding of research that focuses on preventing and treating the underlying causes of cancer.

I am a psychiatrist, not an oncologist. I am an academic physician who has written eight professional books and four books for laypersons. I do my own background research to be as sure as I can that my writing is on solid ground. For this book, I have obtained critical reviews of its technical contents by oncologists and cancer researchers.

I believe that my perspective on oncology from the outside and as a firsthand observer of the best that oncology has to offer gives me the advantage of being free from biases that inevitably accompany being an insider in any field. In this respect, I always have appreciated the views that outsiders have of my own field—psychiatry.

Intriguingly for me, when I talk with oncologists, I find that they turn to me as a psychiatrist and share their frustrations. You can imagine what it is like to be in a medical profession in which the most you can do is try to prolong lives in the face of a lethal disease. Fortunately, they find enough rewards in the patients they treat successfully to keep them going. My overall intent is to support their efforts to improve the outcomes of the patients they serve.

My hope is that my perspective as a person who lives with cancer and as a physician will be useful to you. As a caregiver, I know the ins and outs of receiving the diagnosis of cancer and all that its treatment involves. I know the relief that comes from success and the grief that comes from failure. I know what it is like to go through the process of dying from cancer. I know firsthand both the strengths and the weaknesses of our health care system in general and of cancer care specifically.

Acknowledgements

I am indebted especially to two persons. Philip Krause urged me to write this book and critically reviewed its contents from the point of view of a lay person who wants a detailed, but readable, explanation of what cancer is all about. Jim Koelsch participated in my project by keeping detailed records of his life with advanced cancer to assess the impact of specific treatment and life style changes he has made and by helping me explore the literature on cancer.

In addition to reviewing pertinent literature and the 2011 report *Accelerating Progress against Cancer* and 2012 plan *Shaping the Future of Oncology: Envisioning Cancer Care in 2030* of the American Society of Clinical Oncology both of which concluded that cancer research and care can be vastly improved,[1] I have drawn on the paradigm shifting work of the following authors.

Oncologist Guy Faguet, author of *The War on Cancer: An Anatomy of Failure, A Blueprint for the Future* and the *Conquest of Cancer,*[2] credits the National Cancer Institute (NCI) with "the nation's advances in molecular biology and genetics of cancer." He also criticizes the NCI for "three decades of stagnation in cancer treatment."

Dr. Michael Sporn, professor medicine at the Geisel School of Medicine at Dartmouth and three-decade staff member of the National Cancer Institute, has been struggling for many years to get fellow researchers to think about cancer not as an invasive group of fast-growing cells but as a process, called carcinogenesis (neoplasia). Sporn calls attention to cancer as a multistage process that goes through various cell transformations and sometimes long periods of latency in its progression.[3]

Dr. Siddhartha Mukherjee, author of *The Emperor of All Maladies: A Biography of Cancer*, vividly portrays the history of cancer that culminated with the Cancer Genome Atlas Project.[4] His perspective as an oncologist reveals an insider's view of the past and contemporary state of cancer research and treatment.

In his 2010 *The New Yorker* article "Cancer World: the Making of a Modern Disease," Steven Shapin comprehensively summarized the current state of cancer research and treatment.[5]

In his 2012 book *Cancer as a Metabolic Disease*, Dr. Thomas Seyfried of Boston College makes a compelling case for cancer as a metabolic disease.[6] Seyfried calls the mutations observed in the nuclear DNA of cancer cells "red herrings" that are not the primary causes of neoplasia and consequent origin of cancer cells.

Former executive editor of Fortune magazine, Clifton Leaf expressed outrage over the paltry victories against cancer in his 2004 Fortune magazine article "Why We're Losing The War On Cancer..."[7] He elaborated upon and updated this theme in his 2013 book *The Truth in Small Doses: Why We're Losing the War on Cancer—and How to Win It*.[8] Leaf points out that, although the standardized death rate for cancer in America has fallen, the total number of cancer deaths in the country has risen from 12,500 in 1900 to almost 580,000 in 2013 and by 50% since 1970. That difference is explained largely by our growing and aging population, but it stands in contrast to deaths from heart disease that have fallen by 19% during the same time. Cancer now is the leading cause of death in the world. I have drawn heavily on Leaf's interviews with key persons in the cancer field.

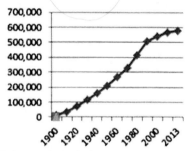

U. S. Annual Deaths from Cancer 1900-2013

Time magazine editor Bill Saporito performed a great public service in his 2013 *Time* article "The Conspiracy to End Cancer" that describes how a team-based, cross-disciplinary approach to cancer research is up-ending tradition and delivering results faster.[9]

The journalist George Johnson set out to learn everything he could about cancer when his wife received that diagnosis at a relatively young age.[10] In his book *The Cancer Chronicles,* he explains that the finely crafted regulators intended to keep cell division in check wear down over time and eventually give way. The result is a cancer cell line whose proliferation gets out of control and, worse, dispatches colonists to other parts of the body.

I am indebted to the generosity of the following professionals for critically reviewing aspects of this book that fall within their areas of expertise: Peter Pedersen, Ph.D., for reviewing the chapter on how cancer cells form and multiply; Douglas McNeel, M.D., Ph.D., for reviewing the chapter on immunotherapy; Dominic D'Agostino, Ph.D., for reviewing the chapter on nutritional therapy and Bharat Aggarwal, Ph.D., David A. Boothman, Ph.D., Gaurab Chakrobarti M.D., Ph.D., Farjana Fattah, Ph.D., Julio Morales, Ph.D., Zachary Moore, M.D., Ph.D., Praveen Patodar, Ph.D. and Ling Xiao, Ph.D. for providing comments as well.

I also am indebted to the following persons who reviewed portions of the book from the perspective of the general reader: James Koelsch, John McCollough, David Williams, Philip Krause, Carolyn Swanson, Steven Swanson and Peter Westman.

Chapter One

Our Journey with Cancer

Why I wrote this book.

I was at a meeting in San Francisco in 1978 and received a call from my wife, Nancy: "Jack, I just came back from our doctor. He said I have a lump in my left breast."

Nancy had a biopsy of the breast lump. It turned out to be cancer—an adenocarcinoma. We were referred to a surgeon who recommended that Nancy have a radical mastectomy. That meant removing her left breast, a muscle underneath it and the lymph nodes from her left armpit—a disfiguring operation. We wondered if that was necessary. Why couldn't he just remove the lump in what is now called a lumpectomy. Her doctor said that he could not be sure that the cancer had not already spread. There was no other way to determine if a few or a lot of cells were in the surrounding tissues or in the lymph nodes. We decided to go ahead with the radical mastectomy.

My curiosity as a physician led me to enquire about research that was going on then regarding the treatment of cancer. I learned about chemotherapy and radiation that were being used to supplement surgery. A few physicians were writing about trying what was called immunotherapy and about nutritional approaches to cancer, but they were in a small minority.

For twenty-six years, there was no evidence that Nancy's cancer had recurred, and I stopped following cancer developments. We felt that she had made the right decision in having a radical mastectomy. Then in 2002

Nancy's physician examined her left breast scar and noticed a lump. That led to removal of the lump and radiation treatment of her left chest. This began the second phase of our life with cancer.

All treatments have predictable or possible side effects. The radical mastectomy was an inconvenience, but a tolerable one. The side effects of the radiation were more than that. Nancy's skin over the radiation site became dry and itching. She developed numbness in her left arm related to damage to her median nerve. As time went on her left hand became clumsy. All of this progressed over the next nine years. But we were grateful Nancy had good health in other respects, and we were content to be followed by our oncologist.

Nancy was supposed to take Tamoxifen for five years, but the side effects were too unpleasant to continue so that she stopped taking it after three years.

In June of 2011, Nancy began to feel short of breath. Over the years, she was an avid walker and had maintained an active life. We went to the emergency room and found that she had fluid in her right pleural space around the lung. Further studies in the hospital revealed that the cancer had recurred and spread from the left chest into the lymph nodes in between the lungs and thence into her right lung. This continued our life with cancer treatment based on the "search for and destroy" model. We now added chemotherapy to surgery and radiation — the triad of conventional cancer treatment.

Nancy had nine pleural fluid drainages. Because of the risk of infection from the pleural taps, a pleurodesis was performed to seal off the pleural space. Because she was not adequately managed with lung expansion exercises after the surgery, she became a pulmonary cripple and needed oxygen continuously for the rest of her life.

Nancy began courses of chemotherapy based on the principle that destroying growing cells would include cancer cells. She lost hair and developed "chemo brain" with a loss of recent memory. At first it looked as though the chemotherapy was shrinking the cancer tumors.

In January of 2012, Nancy required hospitalization from complications of the chemotherapy. She received too much intravenous fluid in the hospital and developed swelling in her legs, which receded with the passage of time.

In June of 2012, it became evident that the chemotherapy was not working, and Nancy entered home-based Hospice Care.

Nancy and I talked about death and dying. It was clear that she did not fear death— only the painful process of dying. We talked about what it would be like at the moment of death and how I had witnessed it twice and was familiar with the literature on the "near death" experience. The first time was with my father when I was in medical school. Dad was in a coma induced by chemotherapy (urethane) for multiple myeloma. I happened to be sitting next to his bed and noticed that his eyes had opened. He stared straight upward for about 30 seconds. Then he smiled, closed his eyes, and stopped breathing. I had the same experience during my internship when I was with a dying woman who also opened her eyes, stared straight upward, closed her eyes and stopped breathing. Nancy and I expressed the hope that we could be together when that time came for her.

Nancy and I reviewed both of our wills and planned our funerals and paid for both of them in advance. We wrote our obituaries, and, since she was an editor, she edited mine. She put the finishing touches on her memoirs entitled *Reminiscences*. We listened to music together. Television no longer held any interest for us. We cherished phone calls and visits from friends and family.

During the last month of her life, Nancy required increasing dosages of morphine to ease the pain of the cancer spreading in her lungs.

On August 31 at 5:00 AM, I was awakened by the sound of Nancy falling out of her hospital bed with side rails. She was in intense pain as I lifted her back into bed. The pain was so great that she pleaded, "Jack, please kill me!" I gave her morphine. We laid together for several hours holding hands. After a while I heard her crying and saw her looking straight up. I asked her if she saw anything. She said "no" with tears.

At around 9:00 AM, I got up and called our hospice team. They came immediately and did what they could to make Nancy comfortable. A volunteer stayed after the hospice nurse left. At 2:14 PM as I was going out the door to get more morphine, she called out to me to come right away. As I approached Nancy, she was looking straight upward. She smiled and stopped breathing at 2:15 PM. I felt a rush of gratitude for being able to be there then. I laid with her holding her hand until the morticians came, crying off and on. They respectfully waited until I felt that I could let Nancy's body go.

For the third time, I had the opportunity to be there at the moment of mortal death and personally witness that moment as reported in the "near death" literature.

Both Nancy and I were most grateful for the Hospice support we received in Florida and Wisconsin. In our view, the nonprofit Hospice systems were the most efficient and compassionate that we encountered during our journey though many medical facilities. The people working in these Hospice systems were clearly dedicated to their work, which they carried out with remarkable empathy and concern for us. This extended into the time when I took advantage of their grief counseling. That experience included reliving and re-enacting my last hours with Nancy.

We had a thirty-four year battle with cancer—or more accurately thirty-four years of living with cancer. Nancy's immune system kept her cancer free for most of her life. In her later years, it failed to recognize cancer cells on two occasions and ultimately became completely blind to them. In one way, we were extremely fortunate. We outlived the usual outcome with breast cancer.

In another way, we lived through an era that lost decades of potential benefit for people with cancer. The focus of cancer funding and research was not on how cancer cells develop and spread. It was on "search for and destroy cancer cells." It was on eliminating cancer cells... not on treating their underlying causes.

In 2013 two of my close relatives were diagnosed with potentially life-threatening cancers.

Conclusion

I have the nagging feeling that, if I had known in 2011 about the complementary therapies for conventional cancer treatment described in Chapter Eleven, Nancy would be living today.

My hope is that our experience will inspire others to take charge of their lives with cancer and become advocates for changing cancer research and care from focusing on killing cancer cells to preventing and stopping neoplasia.

Conventional Cancer Treatment

The conventional surgery/radiation/chemotherapy approach to cancer treatment, its methods and its results are described.

People react to bad news in different ways. The diagnosis of cancer can be emotionally devastating for some who become emotionally debilitated. Others appear to take a cancer diagnosis in stride. Most feel helpless and depend completely on their doctors to direct their treatment. Some are inquisitive and try to learn as much as they can about their particular form of cancer and to do all they can to help their treatment process. The fact that you are reading this book suggests that you are one of them. A few take matters into their own hands and try alternative treatments outside of the conventional cancer care system.

This book is designed to help you understand the basic characteristics of cancer and how to take advantage of the options that are available to you. First of all, the main categories of cancer are:

+ Carcinomas—begin in the skin or in tissues that line or cover internal organs.
+ Sarcomas—begin in bone, cartilage, fat, muscle, blood vessels or other connective or supportive tissue.
+ Leukemias—start in blood-forming tissue, such as bone marrow, and cause large numbers of abnormal blood cells to be produced and enter the blood stream.

+ Lymphoma and myeloma—begin in the cells of the immune system.
+ Central nervous system cancers—begin in the tissues of the brain or spinal cord.

The stages of cancer are:

+ Stage 0 - The earliest, most treatable forms of cancer are when abnormal cells are only detectable in the top layer of cells within the affected body region. Such forms of cancer are often referred to as *carcinoma in situ*, which means that abnormal cells are only located at the site where they originated.
+ Stage I - Abnormal cells clump together and begin penetrating beneath the top layer of cells only within the organ of origin.
+ Stage II - Cancer cells grow into a small tumor within the organ of origin. Typically, cancer in this stage has not spread to other tissues or organs within the body.
+ Stage III - As the cancer tumor grows, cancer cells spread into the lymph nodes and surrounding tissues.
+ Stage IV - Cancer cells spread beyond the surrounding lymph nodes and tissues to other parts of the body. This stage is *metastatic cancer*.

Conventional cancer treatment consists of surgery, radiation, chemotherapy and hormone therapy for some cancers. Surgery and radiation are used to remove or kill cancer cells directly in specific locations. Surgery can result in long-term recovery when a cancer tumor can be completely removed. However, when the cancer cells have gone beyond the original tumor, surgery may facilitate their spread. Targeted radiation techniques, such as multidimensional conformal therapy, intensity-modulated radiation therapy, stereotactic radiosurgery, proton beam radiation therapy and radioimmunotherapy are becoming increasingly available. Brachytherapy involves implanting radioactive pellets, seeds or catheters in or near cancerous tissue.

Chemotherapy and radiation have less positive long-term recovery rates than surgery because they use toxic methods that harm normal cells that divide rapidly—most commonly cells in the bone marrow, digestive tract and hair follicles—and accordingly cannot be used continuously. The most typical side-effects of chemotherapy are myelosuppression (decreased production of white blood cells with suppression of the immune system), mucositis (inflammation of the lining of the digestive tract) and alopecia (hair loss). A patient must recover from these methods before repeating them, and the methods themselves can be carcinogenic, especially radiation. They can kill cancer cells, but those that are not killed continue to grow and spread. This kind of resistance also is seen with the overuse of antibiotics, which creates strains of microbes that are resistant to treatment. Chemotherapy also weakens the immune system, which is the body's natural defense against cancer. This is why chemotherapy and radiation are not seen as cures for cancer.

Because the drugs used to kill cancer cells are toxic to neighboring healthy cells, researchers have long sought a drug delivery method that targets only cancer cells, bypassing the healthy ones. Examples currently available are 1) using Functional Magnetic Resonance Imaging (fMRI) to guide placing drug-filled magnetic nanoparticles in the area of a tumor and 2) using nanoshell particles to protect the enzymes that starve cancer cells as part of chemotherapy.[11] According to the National Cancer Institute, six such nanoparticles are currently approved for use on the market worldwide. So far, they seem to improve the safety of chemotherapy.

Conventional cancer therapy has produced spectacular results. A noteworthy example is Lance Armstrong who survived a battle with cancer that ravaged his testes, lungs and brain. Treatment reduced him to a slip of a man, his bald head scarred by surgery. However, in 1997 he was declared cancer free. Soon thereafter he was cycling up mountains and plunging down their slopes.[12]

Armstrong was treated with Cisplatin—a unique anti-cancer agent. Its development began in the 1960s purely by accident. During an experiment to see what happens to bacteria in electrical fields, it was noticed that the bacteria had stopped multiplying. It seemed they had been poisoned by something that was leaching out of one of the electrodes used to create the electrical field. The substance was identified as platinum. Cisplatin (which contains platinum) was tested against a number of tumors. Overall, it proved of little long-term value, except against testicular cancer, illustrating the fact that no single chemotherapeutic agent in use at this time kills all kinds of cancer cells.

Unfortunately, the general experience with conventional cancer treatment led Ezekiel Emanuel, professor at the University of Pennsylvania School of Medicine, to write a *New York Times* editorial in 2013 on behalf of twenty oncologists critical of the existing cancer care system titled "A Plan To Fix Cancer Care".[13] The editorial stated that many cancer patients, after getting a diagnosis of a frightening disease, pursue any potentially promising therapy regardless of the cost. But the main cost driver is the fee-for-service payment system. The more doctors do for patients, the more reimbursement they receive. Surgeons earn more for every procedure. Oncologists typically make more money if they use newly approved drugs and the latest radiation treatments than if they use cheaper, older alternatives that work just as well. Some of these new therapies are rightly heralded as substantial advances, but others provide only marginal benefit. Of the thirteen anti-cancer drugs the Food and Drug Administration approved in 2012, only one may extend life by more than six months. Two extended life for only four to six weeks. All cost about $6,000 per month of treatment.

The editorial concluded with the statement that we need better incentives for research. Many expensive tests and treatments are introduced without evidence that they significantly improve survival or reduce side effects and with little information about which patients should receive them. For example, while more than 800,000 robotic surgeries, mostly for cancer, were performed from 2011 to 2013, there is no reliable evidence that the robots either improved survival or reduced side effects... despite the fact that they cost more than traditional surgery. Another example is the extent to which major medical centers around the country are spending on genomic analysis equipment before its utility has been demonstrated.

In the same vein, the American Society of Clinical Oncology's (ASCO) 2011 report *Accelerating Progress Against Cancer* concluded that cancer research and care can be vastly improved.[14] It added that, while our understanding of the molecular basis for cancer is growing rapidly, our current approach to developing and testing new therapies is ill-equipped to capitalize on that new knowledge.

The ASCO report went on to say that to realize the greatest potential benefits, the development of treatments should be accompanied by creating diagnostic tests to identify appropriate patients and monitor the outcomes of those treatments in real time. Today, however, diagnostics and treatments are not typically developed and tested at the same time.

ASCO's report added that our approach to cancer has not been based on the fact that all medical interventions depend upon the body's ability to fend off threats to health whether external or internal and on the body's natural healing powers. Instead, the dominant theme has been searching for and destroying cancer tumors by surgery, radiation and chemotherapy. The latter actually interferes with the body's natural defenses and causes mutations in cancer cells that become resistant to treatment.

In 2013, the journalist Alexander Nazaryan spoke with Andrea Hayes-Jordan, a pediatric surgical oncologist at the M. D. Anderson Cancer Center in Houston.[15] She told him that "Our strategic attacks are improving, and we are winning some battles, but not the war yet." Silvia Formenti, who chairs the radiation oncology department at New York University's Langone Medical Center, was even more negative in her assessment of the War on Cancer. She wrote to him in an e-mail, "We have managed to make cancer a huge business, and a national 'terror,' but the progress in reducing mortality is quite questionable."

Preventing Cancer Before It Strikes

In his 2013 book *The Truth in Small Doses: Why We're Losing the War on Cancer-and How to Win It*, Clifton Leaf advocated trying to prevent cancer before it strikes.[16] At Stage 0, a cancerous growth can be detected and removed before it has diversified and spread. By the time a tumor is the size of a grape, it has as many as a billion cells. Those cells become increasingly heterogeneous. Once they break through the membrane that acts as a final barrier between organs and tissues, they are free to spread throughout the body via the bloodstream and/or the lymphatic system.

Leaf finds great promise in chemoprevention pioneered by Dartmouth researcher Michael Sporn, who suggests treating pre-invasive lesions as seriously as full-blown cancers. This seems to fly in the face of the cautious watch-and-wait philosophy popular with many oncologists, who have become convinced (not without reason) that the cure—toxic chemotherapy and high doses of radiation—can be worse than the disease.

However, other than the breast cancer drug tamoxifen and the human papillomavirus (HPV) vaccine—both of which can reduce the risk of getting cancer, not cure it—the promise of chemoprevention remains largely unrealized. A recent article by two preventive oncologists concluded, "There have been numerous chemoprevention trials in the past ten years, but the number of approved chemoprevention drugs is still quite small."[17]

Arguments for Watchful Waiting

A recent study of older men with prostate cancer suggested that "watchful waiting" was often the best route, noting that many patients opted for expensive treatments they didn't need, leading to impotence and incontinence.[18] And a federal task force recommended four years ago that women should delay getting mammograms until age fifty (ten years later than the previous recommendation) because of the procedure's own potential dangers.[19] At the same time, it is advisable for women to learn how to do their own breast examinations as confirmed by a quarter century Canadian study reported in 2014 of women who received either mammograms or did breast examinations and essentially found no difference in death rates.[20]

A group of experts advising the National Cancer Institute (NCI) issued a report recommending that the definition of cancer be changed and that the word cancer be eliminated from some common diagnoses as part of a sweeping change in the nation's approach to cancer detection and treatment.[21] They said, for instance, that some premalignant conditions, like one that affects the breast called "ductal carcinoma in situ" (DCIS), which many doctors agree is not cancer, should be renamed to exclude the word carcinoma so that patients are less frightened and less likely to seek what may be unneeded and potentially harmful treatment that can include the surgical removal of the breast. One way to address the issue is to change the language used to describe lesions found through screening.

According to the NCI group, any lesions detected during breast, prostate, thyroid, lung and other cancer screenings should not be called cancer at all but should instead be reclassified as IDLE conditions, which stands for "indolent lesions of epithelial" origin. "We need a 21st-century definition of cancer instead of a 19th-century definition of cancer, which is what we've been using," said Dr. Otis W. Brawley, chief medical officer for the American Cancer Society.

The impetus behind the call for change is a growing concern among doctors, scientists and patient advocates that hundreds of thousands of men and women are undergoing needless and sometimes disfiguring and harmful treatments for premalignant and cancerous lesions that are so slow growing they are unlikely to ever cause harm.

The advent of highly sensitive screening technology in recent years has increased the likelihood of finding these so-called "incidentalomas"—the name given to incidental findings detected during medical scans that most likely would never cause a problem. However, once doctors and patients are aware a lesion exists, they understandably feel compelled to biopsy, treat and remove it, sometimes at physical and psychological pain and risk to the patient. This is referred to as over-diagnosis, and the resulting unnecessary procedures to which patients are subjected are called over-treatment.

Dr. Larry Norton, a member of the NCI group and Medical Director of the Evelyn H. Lauder Breast Center at Memorial Sloan-Kettering Cancer Center, said the larger problem is that doctors cannot tell patients with certainty which cancers will not progress and which will. "The terminology is just a descriptive term," Dr. Norton said. "But you can't go back and change hundreds of years of literature by suddenly changing terminology."

Still proponents of downgrading cancer with a simple name change say there is precedent for doing so. The NCI report noted that in 1998, the World Health Organization changed the name of an early-stage urinary tract tumor, removing the word "carcinoma" and calling it "papillary urothelial neoplasia of low malignant potential." When a common Pap smear finding called "cervical intraepithelial neoplasia" was reclassified as a low-grade lesion rather than a malignancy, women were more willing to submit to observation rather than wanting treatment then.

"Changing the language we use to diagnose various lesions is essential to give patients confidence that they don't have to aggressively treat every finding in a scan," Dr. Laura Esserman, lead author of the NCI report, said. "The problem for the public is you hear the word cancer, and you think you will die unless you get treated. We should reserve this term, 'cancer,' for those things that are highly likely to cause a problem."

The concern, however, is that since doctors do not yet have a clear way to tell the difference between benign or slow-growing and aggressive tumors, they treat everything as if it might become aggressive. As a result, doctors are finding and treating scores of seemingly precancerous lesions and early-stage cancers—like ductal carcinoma in situ, a condition called Barrett's esophagus, small thyroid tumors and early prostate cancer. But even after years of aggressively treating those conditions, there has not been a commensurate reduction in invasive cancer, suggesting that over-diagnosis and over-treatment are occurring on a significant scale.

Dr. Harold Varmus, Director of the NCI, summarized the situation in 2013 by remarking: "Our investigators are not just looking for ways to detect cancer early, they are thinking about this question of when you find a cancer, what are the factors that might determine how aggressively it will behave. This is a long way from the thinking twenty years ago, when you found a cancer cell and felt you had a tremendous risk of dying."[22]

National Academy of Sciences—Perspective on Cancer Care

The National Academy of Sciences (NAS) provided a comprehensive and authoritative view of contemporary cancer care in 2013.

According to the Committee on Improving the Quality of Cancer

Care of the NAS, more than a decade after the Institute of Medicine first addressed the quality of cancer care in the United States the barriers to achieving excellent care for all cancer patients remain daunting.[23]

The growing demand for cancer care, combined with the complexity of the disease and its treatment, a shrinking workforce and rising costs, constitute a crisis in cancer care delivery. The complexity of cancer impedes the ability of clinicians, patients and their families to formulate plans of care with necessary speed, precision and quality. As a result, decisions about cancer care often are not evidence-based. Many patients also do not receive adequate explanations of their treatment goals, and, when a phase of treatment concludes, they frequently do not know what treatments they have received or the consequences of their treatments for their future health. Many patients also do not have access to palliative care.

Patricia A. Ganz, Chair of the Committee, said that our current cancer care delivery system falls short in terms of consistency that is patient-centered, evidence based and coordinated. She went on to say that if we ignore the signs of crisis in cancer care, we will be forced to deal with an increasingly chaotic and costly system, with exacerbation of existing disparities in the quality of cancer care.

According to Dr. Ganz, oncology care is an extreme example of the best and worst in the health care system today—highly innovative targeted diagnostics and therapeutics alongside escalating costs that do not consistently reflect the value of treatments; tremendous waste and inefficiencies due to poor coordination of care and lack of adherence to evidence-based guidelines with frequent use of ineffective or inappropriate treatments.

The NAS Committee noted that national spending on health care in general currently accounts for 18 percent of the gross domestic product, but it's anticipated to increase to 25 percent by 2037. This rapid growth in health expenditures creates an unsustainable burden on America's economy with far-reaching consequences that will crowd out many national priorities, including investments in education, infrastructure and research; stagnation of employee wages and decreased international competitiveness. In spite of our high health care costs, the United States is in the lowest quartile for life expectancy among countries in the international Organization for Economic Co-operation and Development.

In *U.S. Health in International Perspective: Shorter Lives, Poorer Health*, the Institute of Medicine of the National Academies reported in 2013 that the United States spends far more than other nations on health care in proportion to its earnings as a nation. The $2.6 trillion spent on health care in 2012 is more than twice what we spend on food. About one-third of health care costs are hospitalization expenses—which is more than the United States spends on Social Security ($731 billion) or defense ($718 billion). The United States is among the wealthiest nations in the world, but it is far from the healthiest. For many years, Americans have been dying at younger ages than people in almost all other comparable countries.

Ten percent of the population spends more than 60 percent of our nation's health care costs. These are patients with multiple chronic illnesses and cancer. Other drivers of rising health care costs include the financial incentives of fee-for-service reimbursement that reward volume of care rather than quality or efficiency of care in addition to a lack of coordination and inefficiencies in the health care system.

The multiple reasons for these high costs necessitate a multifaceted solution. The NAS Committee concluded that the fault in the health care system lies with doctors, hospitals, government, insurers, lawyers, patients and their advocacy groups. Everyone is responsible for the American health care dilemma.

Complicating the situation further are the changing demographics in the United States that will place new demands on the cancer care delivery system. The population 65 years and older comprises the majority of patients who are diagnosed with cancer and who die from cancer, as well as the majority of cancer survivors. This population is expected to double between 2010 and 2030. This will result in a 20 percent increase in the number of cancer survivors from 2012 to 2022 and a 45 percent increase in cancer incidence by 2030.

Many cancers are turning into chronic diseases that require more care over a patient's lifetime, further contributing to a rise in cancer care costs. Given the link between obesity and the risk of developing a number of different cancers and other chronic diseases, the growing obesity epidemic is expected to be a driver in rising cancer care costs. In the last 30 years, the obesity rate in adults has doubled, and the childhood obesity rate has more than tripled.

The oncology workforce may soon be too small to care for the growing population of individuals diagnosed with cancer. Studies indicate that cancer care often is not as patient-centered, accessible, coordinated or evidence-based as it could be with a detrimental impact on patients. What's more, advances in understanding the biology of cancer have increased the amount of information a clinician must master to treat cancer appropriately.

Meanwhile, the Centers for Medicare & Medicaid Services, the single largest insurer for this population, is struggling financially as the costs of cancer treatments are escalating unsustainably, making cancer care less affordable for patients and their families and creating disparities in patients' access to high-quality cancer care. The cost of cancer care is rising faster than are other sectors of health care, having increased from $104 billion in 2006 to $125 billion in 2010; costs are expected to increase to $173 billion by 2020. The few tools currently available for improving the quality of cancer care—quality metrics, clinical practice guidelines and information technology—are not widely used and all have serious limitations.

Another driver of cancer care costs are cancer drugs, due in part to their increasing prices. Pharmaceutical companies price these therapies to recoup high research and development costs in addition to profits. As more expensive targeted therapies and other new technologies in surgery and radiation become the standard of care, there are concerns about inappropriate financial incentives in the cancer care system.

The cost of hospital care for cancer patients also is a factor. Hospitals have a negotiating advantage over physicians because they can link bed access and other essential services to their oncology pricing. With this bundling, hospitals can charge more than physicians for chemotherapy treatments despite hospitals' ability to acquire these drugs at a significantly lower cost. UnitedHealthcare figures suggest that hospital markups on drugs average about 250 percent.

Increased cancer care expenditures are not necessarily translating into improvements in cancer outcomes. The median survival for metastatic triple-negative breast cancer is still a little more than one year and is the same or worse in many other major cancers. A lot of cancer care is expensive and offers little for patients. In some cases, it may actually hurt them.

As insurers have decreased their physician payments in order to cut costs, oncologists' revenues have been driven by the profits made on the chemotherapies they administer to their patients. The current fee-for-service reimbursement structure provides an incentive to prescribe more chemotherapy and other expensive treatments even when the patient may not be likely to benefit from them.

The median salary for medical oncologists is $400,000, almost double the salary of most internists. Peter Eisenberg, an oncologist at Marin Specialty Care, noted that in his community practice, six doctors purchase about $8 million worth of chemotherapy each year and sell it for about $10 million. The difference pays their salaries and practice expenses. "Without selling chemotherapy, we wouldn't be in business," he said. "Doctors, like everybody else, respond to incentives."

Hospitals also depend on the earnings from radiation oncology procedures performed on site and encourage their physicians to prescribe such procedures. Reimbursement decisions also influence which radiation procedures physicians order. For example, the rapid adoption of expensive intensity-modulated radiotherapy (IMRT) for prostate cancer replaced much less expensive 3-D conformal radiotherapy, despite limited evidence to support its clinical superiority. From 2001 to 2005, the proportion of patients with non-metastatic prostate cancer who received IMRT increased from 9 percent to 80 percent. By 2008, 95.9 percent of patients received IMRT rather than 3-D conformal radiotherapy. Proton beam therapy, which is even more costly, is now being rapidly implemented.

Patients can face significant financial hardships, such as depleting assets to pay for cancer treatment, going into debt and personal bank-ruptcy. They are poorly informed or have unrealistic expectations about the benefit of interventions and their likelihood of survival. The NAS Committee concluded that the current health care delivery system is poorly prepared to address these concerns comprehensively.

<u>Unrealistic Expectations</u>

In his book *Irrationality in Health Care*, Douglas Hough points out that patients are inclined to poor decision-making when confronted with too many choices and over-optimism that treatments will work without much effort or discomfort on their part.[24] They prefer medication pre-scriptions over life style changes.

Hough points out that, because they're facing a life-threatening ill-ness, cancer patients tend to be inclined to seek treatment regardless of the cost. They aren't going to make rational price-quality/risk trade-offs in purchasing care when they're trying to save their lives. Ninety percent of patients with advanced cancer say that they want to be told the truth about their illness. Still, they often expect to be cured when in fact cure is not possible. One study found that despite having just signed a consent form that stated seven times that their cancer is incurable, one third of patients checked affirmatively on a form that they thought their cancer was curable, and nearly 70 percent thought the goal of the therapy was to get rid of all their cancer.

The unrealistic expectations of patients also are fueled by di-rect-to-consumer marketing. Survival statistics are often quoted in ad-vertisements for health centers, but improvements in survival rates can be misleading because they can include individuals who were over diagnosed or whose cancers may not have required treatment. Physicians also may benefit financially from patients' unrealistic expectations by providing more treatment, even if it is not likely to be effective.

Physicians also can be reluctant to counter patients' unrealistic beliefs about their prognosis because they do not want to make them emotionally distraught or take away their hope. However, studies show that patients who engage in end-of-life care discussions are no more likely to feel worried, sad or distressed than those who do not.

Unrealistic expectations and misaligned financial incentives contribute to the overuse and misuse of interventions in cancer care. Overuse is particularly problematic in individuals with advanced cancer, including treatment with chemotherapy close to the end of life that results in more time spent in the emergency room and the hospital and less time in hospice care. Such aggressive care at the end of life is not helpful for patients and their family members.

One study found that patients receiving more aggressive medical treatment near the end of life had a worse quality of life than those receiving hospice care.[25] Not only is aggressive care near the end of life not in the patient's interests, it's costly. Patients who engaged in end-of-life discussions with their physicians were much less likely to receive aggressive cancer therapy. Another study found palliative care consultation significantly reduced the cost of cancer care.

The Cancer Culture

The National Academy of Sciences Committee on Improving the Quality of Cancer Care suggested that a change in the cancer culture is needed to make cancer care affordable. That culture change will require greater consideration of costs when making health care decisions in addition to balancing the needs of individual patients, physicians, insurers and pharmaceutical companies with the need to improve health care and lower its societal costs. Renzo Canetta, vice president of oncology global clinical research at Bristol-Myers Squibb, said that there is a need to recognize that "we are all in the same type of boat, even though we may have different employers. Progress is going to come only from collaboration and not from creating little parishes where we fight against each other on petty issues."

Clinicians need to realistically convey to patients their prognoses; the costs, potential benefits and side effects of various treatment options and palliative care and end-of-life care considerations. Drug labels or consent forms provide information on risks and side effects, but rarely provide information on expected benefits that is quantified and tailored to a patient and to his or her comorbidities. The way chemotherapies are labeled and consent forms are written should provide clear, simple and direct statements about the expected magnitude of benefit from the treatment. They should provide the percentage of patients still living 1 or 2 years after treatment.

The American Society of Clinical Oncology has undertaken an effort to change the cancer culture through its Quality Oncology Practice Initiative (QOPI). The QOPI is a practice-based quality improvement program developed by practicing oncologists and quality experts, using clinical guidelines and published standards.[26] The goal of QOPI is to promote excellence in cancer care by helping practices create a culture of self-examination and improvement.

The QOPI assesses performance and then provides feedback and improvement tools for hematology and oncology practices to improve the quality of cancer care. Some of the QOPI performance metrics include having a discussion with a patient about the intent of chemotherapy, providing a patient with a chemotherapy treatment plan and providing appropriate hospice enrollment. However, only less than 10 percent of oncology practices in the United States currently employ the QOPI. In addition, few QOPI-certified practices are maintained at academic medical centers where future oncologists undergo training.

Separating cancer specialists' income from treatment choices is important. The fees for radiologic procedures help pay for physicians' salaries, and also help reimburse the costs of the hospital or other facility that owns the radiology equipment. Instead provider incentives should be aligned toward patient-centered, coordinated care among cancer specialists, such as radiologists, medical oncologists and primary care physicians. This would improve the information patients have to make decisions about and manage their care. Effective communication is a key component of effective cancer care. Communication across cultures can be challenging, especially if there are language barriers.[27] Clinicians should be reimbursed for communication with patients, including provision of accurate information on a patient's prognosis; the costs, potential benefits and side effects of various treatment options; end of life planning and palliative and hospice care considerations.

Conclusion

After getting the diagnosis of a frightening disease, many cancer patients pursue any potentially promising therapy, regardless of the cost. They may receive expensive tests and treatments without evidence that they improve survival or reduce side effects and with little information about whether or not it is appropriate for them. Fortunately, most receive the best care available today, and many significantly extend their life expectancies...some dramatically.

According to the Committee on Improving the Quality of Cancer Care of the National Academy of Sciences, more than a decade after the Institute of Medicine first addressed the quality of cancer care in the United States the barriers to achieving excellent care for all cancer patients remain daunting. The current health care delivery system is poorly prepared to address these concerns comprehensively.

To achieve the greatest potential benefits, the development of cancer treatments should be accompanied by creating diagnostic tests to identify appropriate patients and monitor the outcomes of those treatments in real time. Today diagnostics and treatments are not typically developed and tested at the same time.

Even with the insights arising from the shortcomings of conventional cancer treatment and the increasing application of immunotherapy, there likely will not be simple cures as once envisaged. Still many kinds of cancer could be transformed from killers into manageable conditions. Then neoplasia would become something to live with, just as people now live with diabetes, cardiovascular disease or even HIV.

Navigating the Cancer Care System

This chapter shows how the information in this book can be used by persons receiving cancer care and their caregivers to become more personally and authoritatively involved in decisions that confront them. The Introduction is for reading now. The remainder of the chapter is for later reference.

Introduction

For everyone, the key to preventing and living with cancer optimally is taking responsibility for your own health. If you do not have cancer or are a caregiver, it means keeping physically and emotionally fit with a positive outlook on life and doing what you can to prevent cancer in yourself. If you have cancer, it means doing everything you can to understand and manage your particular form of cancer. This involves:

+ doing research to build your own expertise about maintaining your own health and understanding your medical conditions;
+ keeping your own health records so that you will have them readily accessible and so that you can follow your own progress or lack of it;
+ keeping abreast of the latest developments regarding your medical problems that your doctors may not have time to follow;

+ knowing what questions to ask your doctors and when to get a second opinion; and
+ becoming an expert about your own medical problems.

In essence, you need to know as much as you can about yourself. Although it may be easier to simply rely on your health care professionals to take care of you, there's no one who cares more about you than you do. Actually, being an expert on your own health and medical problems is empowering. It's the most effective way to ensure that you will receive the best health care and results possible.

If you have cancer or are a caregiver, subsequent chapters in this book give you a foundation for raising questions with your doctors about your care and what can be done to make the most effective and manageable decisions. The most important questions for you are:

+ What cell type of cancer do I have?
+ How aggressive are the cancer cells?
+ What diagnostic tests do I need?
+ What are the forms of treatment available to me?
+ What outcome can I expect from each form of treatment?
+ What are the side effects of each treatment?
+ What is my life expectancy according to studies of my kind of cancer?
+ Will my insurance cover required treatments?
+ Is there a clinical trial that I should consider entering?
+ What do you know about the cause of my form of cancer?
+ Should I obtain a second opinion?

If you have specific questions, medical specialty societies representing more than 500,000 physicians developed a list of *Five Things Physicians and Patients Should Question* for a range of specific conditions and circumstances to stimulate doctor/patient conversations that will improve care and eliminate unnecessary tests and procedures.[1] These lists include specific recommendations physicians and patients should discuss to help make wise decisions about the most appropriate care based on their individual situation. Each list provides information on when specific tests and procedures may be appropriate.

You can expect that your doctors are like any other professionals and are not able to keep up with all of the information that you can access about your form of cancer, especially alternative, naturalistic therapies. You will need to make your own judgments about your options. This book gives you a foundation for making appropriate enquiries and decisions for yourself.

You and your doctors are confronted with uncertainties, and your interests are not well served by waiting until research reveals answers to your questions that become accepted medical practices. A guiding principle is that using all of the resources and remedies available to you will help to ensure that you are not missing something that could benefit you. This especially is the case with nutritional approaches that have not been adopted by mainstream medicine but that are not harmful and possibly could help you.

The best way to be on top of your health care is to keep your own records, both for their accessibility and for giving you background for asking questions and doing your own research.

If you have read this far in this book, my guess is that you are motivated to become an expert on your own health with the help of your professionals. Still you may want to skip or skim the rest of this chapter because it goes into more detail than you need right now if your primary interest is learning more about how to manage cancer. I have placed this information early in the book to emphasize its importance because it is the foundation of effectively living with cancer, but you may wish to return to it later when it is more relevant to your current interests.

Electronic Hospital and Clinic Records

Your health care system keeps electronic records on all of its patients. There is a national organization, the Healthcare Information and Management Systems Society (HIMSS), that leads efforts to optimize health care by using information technology. The HIMSS Electronic Health Record Association (EHRA) is a trade association of electronic health record companies that addresses national efforts to create inter-operable Electronic Health Records (EHRs) in hospital and clinic settings.[2] The EHRA operates on the premise that the rapid, widespread adoption of EHRs will help improve the quality of patient care as well as the productivity and sustainability of the health care system itself. The EHRA's Code of Conduct encourages cooperative and transparent business practices among industry stakeholders, including responsible development; patient safety; interoperability and data portability; clinical and billing accuracy, privacy and security and patient engagement.

Unlike paper-based records that require manual control, EHRs are secured by technological tools. There are three kinds of technology that can improve the security and permanence of electronic records:

- Deterrents–These focus on the ethical behavior of people and include controls such as alerts, reminders and education of users. Another useful form of deterrent is Audit Trails. This system records the identity, times and circumstances of users accessing information. If system users are aware of such a record keeping system, it discourages them from taking ethically inappropriate actions.

- Technological obstacles–These directly control the ability of users to access information and ensure that they only access information they need to know according to their job requirements. Examples of technological obstacles include authorization, authentication, encryption and firewalls.

- System management precautions–This involves proactively monitoring the information system to ensure that known sources of vulnerability are eliminated, such as with antivirus and fire-wall software.

- External hard disc or cloud backup of your computer files.

The extent of information security concerns about electronic records goes beyond these technical issues. Each transfer of information from your health care system to anyone else must be authorized by you.

SeeYourChart

Through SeeYourChart (also known as SeeMyChart) both you and your doctors have read-only access to your electronic medical summaries, lab results, appointment calendar and patient education.[3] SeeYourChart is easy to use so you can use it no matter what your computer skills might be. However, since health care facilities set the criteria for what you can see and when it is available to you, SeeYourChart is not a personal health record that you can control. You can authorize access for family members, caregivers and other physicians, thereby improving communication about, and understanding of, your status and treatment.

Epic MyChart

Epic is a major provider of medical information systems.[4] If your health care provider uses an Epic medical record system, the Epic Integrated Personal Health Record MyChart gives you access, via browser or mobile app (for iOS and Android) to the same records your doctor use. Not all Epic MyChart functions are available on mobile and are changing in capabilities. You can:

- View test results
- View upcoming & past appointments
- Fill out pre-visit questionnaires
- Schedule appointments
- View paperless statements & pay bills online
- Upload photos
- Update medications and allergies
- Connect to home devices
- Refill prescriptions
- Message securely with providers
- View a child's records and print growth charts
- Manage the care of elderly parents
- View education topics triggered by your data

     ✦ Get a chronic disease summary with reminders

The Personal Health Record (PHR)

The best way to understand and keep track of your health is by maintaining your own Personal Health Record (PHR) that you control yourself.[5] A PHR provides you with a complete and accurate summary of your medical history and information that is available to you whenever you need it. Your PHR can be on paper, electronic or both. Examples of personal electronic health records are My Medical, Personal Portable Electronic Medical Record and Epic Lucy. Your primary care or oncology record office can advise you as to which of these forms of electronic software fits best with its electronic record system.

Before starting a PHR it is worthwhile to think about its downside. One of the most controversial issues for PHRs is how technology could threaten the privacy of your information. Network computer break-ins are becoming more common. Thus storing medical information online outside of your control and even in your own computer can risk the exposure of your health information to unauthorized individuals. At the same time, this possibility already exists with the electronic records used in health care facilities. This is why they require your written consent to transmit information about you to others. For most of us, the possibility of unauthorized use of our electronic medical records is not a significant issue if we take the usual precautions to protect our computers.

Epic Lucy

Unlike the Epic MyChart, the Epic PHR Lucy is not connected to any facility's electronic medical record system.[6] It stays with you wherever you receive care and allows you to organize your medical information in one readily accessible place. You can request an updated electronic copy of your medical record and store it in Lucy. You also can add information about your health and share it with other places where you receive care. You can enter health data directly into Lucy, pull in MyChart data or upload standards-compliant Continuity of Care Documents from other facilities. Epic's Care Everywhere software also can retrieve documents from Lucy, making this information available to clinicians as part of the electronic chart.

If your insurance changes or you move and leave your current health care organization, Lucy will follow you.

Epic Lucy is only available through health care providers as an off-shoot of a MyChart system. Your health care provider can tell you how to set up an Epic Lucy PHR or their own electronic equivalent that is an extension of their MyChart. Once it is set up Lucy is portable. Its functionality is evolving over time.

ASCO Cancer Treatment Summaries

An American Society of Clinical Oncology (ASCO) Cancer Treatment Plan and Summary provides a convenient way to store information about your cancer, cancer treatment and follow-up care.[7] It's meant to give basic information about your medical history to any doctors who will care for you during your lifetime. Using the treatment summary, your current oncologist can enter the chemotherapy dose you received, the specific drugs that were used, the number of treatment cycles that were completed, surgeries done and any additional treatment that was given, such as radiation therapy or hormonal therapy.

ASCO also offers a form called a Survivorship Care Plan based on specific clinical practice guidelines for certain types of cancer.[8] This document guides your follow-up care after cancer treatment is finished.

AccessMyRecords

Preventable medical errors are the fifth leading cause of death in the U.S. Yet 93 percent of those errors could have been avoided if the doctor or emergency responder had access to a personal health record or medical summary of the patient at the time of the initial treatment. Access My Records is an internet based PHR service that provides simple, secure and confidential cloud storage for its member's crucial health, medical and legal records.[9] Using AccessMyRecords.com, you can file and manage your personal health records and then access them, whenever or wherever needed, via any internet connected computer or smartphone by using the Company's AMR–ICE (In Case of Emergency) Program. No special software or hardware is necessary, and your information will remain confidential.

Emergency responders now are trained to look for a personal ID or medical ID card upon arrival at the scene. An Access My Records ID Card in your wallet, a Key Tag on your key ring and Window Decals for your car or home will not be overlooked and will enable emergency personnel to have instant access to your personal and medical records, vital information that could help save your life.

Advance Directives

After preparing or updating your last will and testament with your attorney, the first consideration is about the kind of medical care you want if you are too ill or injured to express your wishes. Advance Directives are legal documents that allow you to spell out your decisions about end-of-life care ahead of time. They give you a way to tell your family, friends and health care professionals about your wishes and to avoid confusion later on.

Even if you are in good health now, you should write an Advance Directive. By creating an Advance Directive, you're making your preferences about medical care known before you're faced with a serious injury or illness. An accident or serious illness can happen suddenly, and if you already have a signed Advance Directive, your wishes are more likely to be followed. You may want to plan, and even pay for, your own funeral. There is a financial benefit in paying for your funeral in advance by locking in the cost at current price levels. These preparations will spare your loved ones the need to make critical decisions about your care while you are incapacitated and at the time of your death.

Any adult can prepare an Advance Directive that does not have to be a complicated legal document. It can contain short, simple statements about what you want done or not done if you can't speak for yourself. Remember, anything you write by yourself or with a computer software package should follow your state laws. You also may want to have what you have written reviewed by your doctor or a lawyer to make sure your specific directives are understood exactly as you intended. When you are satisfied with your Directive, it should be notarized, and copies should be given to your family and your doctor.

You may change or cancel your Advance Directive at any time, as long as you are considered of sound mind, which means that you are able to think rationally and communicate your wishes in a clear manner. Again, your changes must be made, signed and notarized according to the laws in your state. Make sure that your doctor and any family members who know about your Directive also are aware that you have changed it and where it is currently located.

You can write an Advance Directive in the following ways:

+ Use a form provided by your doctor.
+ Write down your wishes yourself.
+ Contact your health department or state department on aging to get a form.
+ Contact a lawyer.
+ Use an internet software package for legal documents.

An Advance Directive includes a living will, a durable power of attorney for health care and a do not resuscitate order. If included in one document, it must be properly witnessed, preferably by a notary of the public. If in separate documents, each one must be properly witnessed or notarized.

<u>What is a living will?</u>

A living will is a written legal document that describes the kind of medical treatments or life-sustaining treatments you do or do not want if you are seriously or terminally ill. You might include instructions on:

- Organ or tissue donation
- The use of dialysis and breathing machines
- Tube feeding

A living will doesn't include selecting someone to make decisions for you.

What is a durable power of attorney for health care?

A durable power of attorney (DPA) for health care enables you to choose others to make health care decisions for you. It becomes active any time you are unconscious or unable to make medical decisions. A DPA allows a trusted person to carry out your wishes in your living will in situations that require making judgments. But a DPA may not be a good choice if you don't have another person you can trust to make these decisions for you.

Living wills and DPAs are legal documents in most states. Even if they aren't officially recognized by law in your state, they can still guide your loved ones and doctors when you are unable to make decisions about your medical care.

What is a do not resuscitate order?

A do not resuscitate (DNR) order is specific kind of advance directive. A DNR is a request to not have cardiopulmonary resuscitation (CPR) if your heart stops or if you stop breathing. Unless given other instructions, health care workers will try to help anyone whose heart has stopped beating or who has stopped breathing. You can specify in your Advance Directive that you don't want to be resuscitated. Your doctor will put the DNR order in your medical chart. Doctors and hospitals in all states accept DNR orders.

Talk with your family as well as doctors and others close to you about the specifics of your Advance Directive and make sure they are readily available.

The Costs of Cancer Care

Dr. Peter Ubel, professor of medicine at Duke University, advises patients to enquire about the costs of cancer care since their insurance may not fully cover it.[10] He points out that the financial burden of paying for medical care can cause more distress than many medical side effects. For example The Center for American Progress estimates that a breast-cancer patient in Massachusetts with a high deductible plan could face more than $50,000 in medical expenses.

As people live longer with terminal diseases, the costs associated with their care rise. The risk often is not just that there will not be enough money to provide that care, but that a surviving spouse will be left alone and destitute. With health care advisers cautioning that terminal care expenses could rise to $1 million or more for the last years of life, they say there are simple and sophisticated strategies to make the most of the money at hand for those with savings and foresight.[11] Often people find themselves making financial decisions based on emotions, short-term urgency and on misinformation.

Under emotional duress, caregivers suffer declines in health themselves, take time off from work or quit entirely and lose income. They may fail to save money or tend to their own portfolios. Good advice can make a difference when people have assets to pay for two to four years of care. One strategy is to lay out the best and worst cases for how long someone is going to live and how sick that person is likely to get. From that, a range of costs can be determined.

The reality is that most people with a long-term disease requiring palliative care will quickly become dependent on public benefits. "People think Medicare will cover all their costs, but it's very minimal for long-term care," said Jed Levine, executive vice president and director for programs and services at the Alzheimer's Association's New York chapter. "It's 100 days in a nursing home for rehabilitation. It's not custodial care."

Medicaid is intended to provide health care to people who are indigent, including those who are disabled or elderly. Paying for long-term care at home or in a nursing facility is an effective way to quickly run out of money. The national median rate for a year in a nursing home is $83,950. In New York State, it is $125,732.[12]

The exact qualifications for Medicaid vary by state and will continue to do so. Most states now will cover nursing home expenses for someone whose income is $2,100 or less each month and who has $2,000 or less in assets, not including the primary residence. The threshold is substantially lower for at-home care. In New York the monthly income limit for receiving care at home is $800 or $1,175 for a couple. Any surplus that materializes must be spent on the patient's care for that person to remain eligible. New York's home care program requires that a person cannot have more than $14,400 in savings—or $21,150 for a couple—but retirement accounts of any value are exempt with the exception of distributions that do count as income.

Most people would prefer that their family inherit their life savings. But if in the five years before applying for Medicaid, a person transfers any assets—for example, money or property to children or grandchildren—the giver would incur a penalty upon enrollment. Those five years are known as the look-back period.

There are a handful of exceptions. Federal law keeps some assets out of the equation altogether. A patient's house is exempt, if the equity in it falls under a threshold that varies by state from $500,000 to $802,000, and if the enrollee plans to remain there or to return after a stay elsewhere for medical care. Personal belongings are also exempt, like furniture or even a car. So are small life insurance policies and prepaid funerals.

Since the late 1980s, federal laws have included protections against "spousal impoverishment," allowing the healthy spouse to retain a modest income—depending on the state of residency, currently up to $1,938 to $2,989 each month—without affecting the ill spouse's Medicaid eligibility. Spousal protection laws also allow the healthy spouse to keep half the couple's assets, as much as $115,920 in some states and as little as $22,000 in others.

One strategy, called pooled trusts, has become more popular in the states where it's available. Pooled trusts, run by nonprofit organizations, allow the elderly or disabled to maintain more of their income and assets than Medicaid otherwise permits. Participants submit their income each month to a special trust managed by a third party. The trust pays the participant's basic living expenses, including rent or mortgage payments and utilities. Still, registering for a trust is complicated. Experts recommend that families seek help from experienced professionals when applying for Medicaid. Mistakes can cost thousands of dollars and incur penalties that will reduce coverage.

End of life planning requires thoughtful consideration of the costs involved. Advice regarding federal and state benefits can be obtained from the Center for Medicaid and for veterans from the Department of Veterans Affairs.[13]

An Argument for Life Panels

Bob Goldman, a financial planner, told the story of his mother in a New York Times article.[14] At the beginning of 2012 his mother was 95 years old. She lived in an assisted-living center with hospice care in a hospital bed 24/7. She was hollow-eyed and emaciated. Though she had moments of clarity, she was confused, anxious and uncomfortable. Her quality of life was minimal, at best. And the cost to keep her in this condition had risen to close to $100,000 a year.

Three years earlier, when she was completely rational, Bob's mother told him that she had lived a full and rewarding life and was ready to go. By 2012, when her life was more punishment than reward, she did not have the mental faculties to reaffirm her desire, nor was there a legal way to carry out her decision. Even if she had been living in one of the states like Oregon, Washington or Montana that have "death with dignity" procedures, the fact that she lacked mental competency to request an assisted death in 2012 almost certainly would have ruled out any possibility that her wish would be granted.

Nor would it have been an option to move her to one of the few countries that have removed the legal perils of a decision to end one's life. It was hard enough to get his mother from her bed to her chair. How would he have transported her to Belgium, Switzerland or the Netherlands?

Goldman believes that there is only one solution for this type of situation. What is needed here, he suggests, is a "life panel" with the legal authority to ensure that his mother's request to end her own life, on her own terms, would be honored.

Goldman is staking a claim on the name "life panel" because the concept of "death panels" has been so irresponsibly bandied about during debates about the government's involvement in health care.

The financial aspects of the end of life are an integral part of almost every plan Goldman creates in his professional work. Some of Goldman's clients are realistic about the crushing expenses they could face in their final years. Others are more sanguine. When he tells them that their money is unlikely to last through their 90s, they say: "Well, that's O.K. I don't plan to live past 85, anyway." Goldman has a standard answer in these cases. He says: "Yes, you expect to die at 85, but what if you're unlucky? What if you live to 95? At that point, I tell them about my mother. Then we get down to work."

Occasionally, people tell Goldman that their end dates are guaranteed. They are saving pills that will put them out of their misery, or they have made "arrangements" with friends. For all their planning, these persons do not realize that when the time comes, they may be too sick or demented to carry out their do-it-yourself strategies. And so he comes back to the life panel. Who is on it? Certainly, a doctor would be involved. After all, we laypersons might feel guilty about making decisions that would hasten the end of a life, but doctors would be guilty of murder under current law in most states. On a statutory life panel, a doctor would be held blameless. And Goldman would have no problem adding a medical ethicist and a therapist.

Most importantly, he thinks an individual should be allowed to nominate panelists who are likely to understand the person's wishes: family members, close friends or a person with whom they share religious beliefs.

A "life panel" may seem like a reach, but in fact we already come quite close to this now with Advance Directives. But legal documents only go so far. Doctors know firsthand the uncertainties of deciding when a person has lost medical decision-making capacity. Nor is it possible to write out instructions for every possible medical eventuality. A life panel might not be the perfect solution, but neither is draining a family's resources to support a joyless existence in a hospital bed.

The American Medical Association and the Institute of Medicine have recommended that end of life "advance care planning" be a reimbursable by health insurance programs.[15]

Readings on Cancer Care

The American Cancer Society provides a list of a variety of books on cancer, largely devoted to its specific forms.[16]

The National Cancer Institute also offers a list of a number of books dealing with cancer and cancer-related topics.[17]

The American Psychosocial Oncology Society offers books that deal with family, emotional and practical issues related to cancer and caregivers.[18]

Oncologist-sponsored information about cancer can be obtained from the American Society of Clinical Oncology.[19]

Dr. Peter Ubel offers advice on how to get the most out of your health care in his book *Critical Decisions: How You and Your Doctor Can Make the Right Medical Choices Together*.[20] He gives you background information about how doctors think and work.

After twelve years, sixteen cancer occurrences and counting, Lorie L. Vincent and her husband Mark chronicled their approach to living and thriving during years of suffering. In their book *Fighting Disease, Not Death*, they go beyond the relentless progression of the disease to describe the anchoring faith that sustains them and gives them a reason to remain in service to others.[21] They compare their decision to fight disease and not worry about the moment of death to approaches others take when faced with lifelong suffering.

In their book *The Good Fight* psychologist Greg Holmes and physician Katherine Roth go well beyond their personal struggle for survival when confronted by cancer.[22] They offer a hard-hitting critique of currently accepted mainstream cancer therapies. They put self-advocacy as being possibly the most powerful therapy of all.

Madhulika Sikka's book *A Breast Cancer Alphabet* offers a new way to live with and plan for the hardest diagnosis that most women will ever receive.[23] It is a personal, practical and deeply informative look at the road from diagnosis to treatment and beyond. It goes where many fear to tread.

The Professional Patient Advocate Institute is a resource for practitioners who want to enhance, elevate and improve their skills in the burgeoning field of patient advocacy.[24] It exists to help professional advocates navigate the increasingly complex world of healthcare and empowering patients in order to create a culture of patient- and family-centeredness and improving health care quality.

The book *ABC of Cancer Care* is a practical primary care guide to help health professionals better inform their patients, manage and recognize the common complications of cancers and their treatment, and understand the rationale and implications of decisions made in secondary and tertiary care.[25]

The Alternative Cancer Research Institute has published *The Complete Guide to Alternative Cancer Treatment* as a resource for exploring treatments that can be used separately or in conjunction with conventional treatments.[26]

Conclusion

For everyone, the key to preventing and living with cancer is taking responsibility for your own health. If you do not have cancer or are a caregiver, it means keeping physically and emotionally fit with a positive outlook. In essence, you need to know as much as you can about yourself. Actually, being an expert in your own health and medical problems is empowering. It's the most effective way to ensure that you will receive the best health care possible.

Your health care system keeps electronic records on all of its patients. Unlike paper-based records that require manual control, electronic health records are secured by technological tools. You can gain read-only access to your electronic medical summaries, lab results, appointment calendar and patient education through SeeYourChart, also known as

SeeMyChart. The best way to understand and keep track of your health is by keeping a Personal Health Record (PHR) that you control yourself.

Advance Directives are legal documents that allow you to spell out your decisions about end-of-life care ahead of time. They give you a way to tell your family, friends and health care professionals about your wishes and to avoid confusion later on. They include a living will, a durable power of attorney for health care and a do not resuscitate order.

The costs associated with medical and nursing home care during terminal illnesses can be devastating. You are well-advised to enquire and keep track of the costs of cancer care since your insurance most likely will not fully cover it. Being aware of Medicare and Medicaid benefit limitations is important. The financial burden of paying for medical care can cause more distress than many medical side effects. This is especially the case with rehabilitation and nursing home care that has limited insurance coverage.

Often people find themselves making financial decisions based on emotions, short-term urgency and on misinformation. Instead there are simple and sophisticated strategies to make the most of the money at hand for those with savings and foresight.

There are a number of books and publications that can be helpful in understanding and managing your own health and your medical problems.

Background for Understanding Cancer

The history of cancer and the development of cancer care are reviewed to offer you a broad perspective on cancer.

I found Steven Shapin's 2010 *The New Yorker* article, "Cancer World: The Making of a Modern Disease" to be an excellent overview of cancer extending back over at least 120,000 years.[1] Dating back to that time, a bone tumor cavity was discovered in the rib of a Neanderthal found in present-day Croatia. "Normally ribs are full of spongy bone, but this rib has a big cavity," said David W. Frayer, an anthropologist at the University of Kansas. He added, "People didn't live as long then, and they weren't exposed to carcinogens as they are today. This shows that they were susceptible to cancer as we are today, even in a non-polluted environment."

Before this discovery, the earliest known bone cancers were found in specimens 1,000 to 4,000 years old. An Egyptian papyrus from about 1600 B.C. described tumors of the breast and concluded: "There is no treatment." The Greeks made a distinction between benign tumors (oncos) and malignant ones (carcinos). What plagued Atossa, the ancient Persian queen who is believed to have suffered from breast cancer, still plagues us today.

In the second century A.D., Galen reckoned that the cause of cancer was systemic, an excess of melancholy or black bile, one of the body's four "humors," brought on by bad diet and environmental circumstances.

Ancient medical practitioners sometimes cut tumors out, but the prognosis was known to be grim.

Shapin notes that cancer has always been with us, but not always in the same way. Its care and management have differed over time, of course, but so, too, have its identity, visibility, meanings and frequency. Pick up the thread of history at its most distant end and you have cancer the crab—so named either because of the spreading out of a tumor or because its pain is like the pinch of a crab's claw.

The experience of cancer has always been terrible, but, until modern times, its effect on our society has been light. In the past, the common fear was of dying from other causes: infectious diseases (plague, smallpox, cholera, typhus, typhoid fever); "apoplexies" (what we now call strokes and heart attacks); and, most notably in the nineteenth century, "consumption" (tuberculosis). The agonizing manner of cancer death was dreaded, but that fear was not centrally situated in the public mind—as it now is. This is one reason that the medical historian Roy Porter wrote that cancer is "the modern disease par excellence," and that Siddhartha Mukherjee calls it "the quintessential product of modernity."

A Disease of Civilization?

Shapin found that at one time cancer was seen as a "disease of civilization," belonging to much the same causes as "neurasthenia" and diabetes, the former a nervous weakness believed to be brought about by the stress of living and the latter a condition produced by "bad diet and indolence."

In the eighteenth and nineteenth centuries, some physicians attributed cancer—notably of the breast and the ovaries—to psychological and behavioral causes. William Buchan's wildly popular eighteenth-century text *Domestic Medicine* judged that cancers might be caused by "excessive fear, grief, or religious melancholy."[2] In the nineteenth century, reference was repeatedly made to a "cancer personality," and, in some versions, specifically to sexual repression. Cancer was considered shameful, not to be mentioned...even obscene. Among the Romantics and the Victorians, suffering and dying from tuberculosis might be considered a badge of refinement; dying from cancer was not.

Cancer is "the modern disease" not just because we understand it in new ways but also because there's much more cancer around. For some cancers, the rise in incidence is clearly connected with things that get into our bodies that once did not. The link between smoking and lung cancer is the most clear-cut example. But Shapin sees the rise in cancer mortality, in a macabre way, as good news: as we live longer, and as many infectious diseases have ceased to be major causes of death, we have become prone to maladies that express themselves at ages once uncommonly attained.

In the middle of the nineteenth century the life expectancy in the United States was less than 40; at the beginning of the twentieth century, it was 47 years. Now the median age at diagnosis for breast cancer in the United States is 61; for prostate cancer it's 67; and for colorectal cancer it's 70. In the United States, about half of all men and about a third of all women will contract cancer in their lifetimes. In 2013 cancer ranked just below heart disease as the cause of death in the United States. But in poor countries with shorter life expectancies, it doesn't even make the top ten.

Siddhartha Mukherjee, an oncologist and the author of *The Emperor of All Maladies*, wrote a history of the disease and of the attempts to describe it, explain it, manage it, cure it or just to reconcile its victims to their fate.[3] He wrote a personal account of his own "coming-of-age as an oncologist." He is sure that he can do much more for his patients than the physicians of the past, yet he knows that he shares many of their frustrations. At the same time, he wants to understand what his patients have in common with their ailing forebears and what is peculiarly modern about their predicament. He sees cancer as a world unto itself. As one victim of sarcoma told Mukherjee, "I am in the hospital even when I am outside the hospital."

Mukherjee notes that the cancers of the past were visible on the body's surface; now we have visual access through advances in microscopy, tissue staining, biopsies, X-rays, positron emission tomography (PET), computed tomography (CT) and magnetic resonance imaging (MRI). All of these have given us new possibilities for understanding cancer...and a new vocabulary of fear.

In his book *The Illness Narrative*, the psychiatrist and anthropologist Arthur Kleinman recorded conversations between cancer victims and their physicians.[4] A dying patient with metastasized rectal cancer told his doctor about his feeling that "there is something not me in me, an 'it', eating its way through the body. . . . These cancer cells are me and yet not me"...an accurate description of cancer.

In 1957 Frank Burnet, the Nobel Prize winning Australian microbiologist, studied the ability of our bodies to distinguish 'self' from 'non-self', meaning that an immune response is only mounted against 'non-self' molecules, while 'self' molecules are ignored by our immune systems.[5] He pointed out that in cancer the immune system fails to do its job to eliminate cancer cells. At the University of Melbourne, he wrote about immunology, particularly autoimmunity and the immune surveillance of cancer. Because he saw cancer as resulting from malfunctioning of his body, he was not optimistic about finding a cure for it. He ultimately died of colon cancer at the age of 86.

In 1963 Dr. Joseph H. Burchenal of the Memorial Sloan-Kettering Institute for Cancer Research pointed out that "it is unlikely that chemotherapeutic agents against cancer will be any more effective, unless there is some sort of an active immunological response that can be evoked."[6] Antibiotics reduce the number of bacteria, but our immune systems are needed to cure the diseases they cause. The same principle applies to chemotherapy and cancer cells.

In the 1970s cancer was being recognized as a multifaceted process. As time went on the diversity of cancer became more evident. Just knowing that all cancers were malignant tumors was not enough.

In 1982, Dr. Lewis Thomas described *immunosurveillance* as a primary defense mechanism against cancer in human beings. He brought out the way white blood cells act as sentinels in recognizing and eliminating continuously arising aberrant cells. He added that this mechanism may play a somewhat different role in humans than in most experimental animal models.[7] Dr. Thomas, former head of the Memorial Sloan-Kettering

Cancer Center, suffered from a rare form of cancer named after one of his friends, Jan Waldenstrom of Sweden, and died in 1993 at the age of 80.

Progress in cancer care was along the lines of discovering that lumpectomies (removal of the tumor) were as effective as radical mastectomies. William Stewart Halsted began to perform radical mastectomies at Johns Hopkins Hospital in the eighteen-nineties. They were called "radical" because the aim was to remove the "root" of cancers. Disdainful of what he called "mistaken kindness," Halsted proceeded to excavate more and more tissue—digging out the muscles of the breast cavity along with the lymph nodes and glands above and underneath the collar bone. Over time, surgeons learned more about what to cut out and what to leave. The far less extensive "lumpectomy" operation for breast cancer, pioneered in the nineteen-twenties by the English surgeon Geoffrey Keynes, was given its name as a sneer by American Halstedians...it seemed insufficiently aggressive. But by the nineteen-eighties it was accepted that outcomes among patients receiving "simple mastectomies" were statistically identical to those for patients undergoing the radical operation.

The *Journal of the National Cancer Institute* reported that progress in cancer research in the 1980s ranged from basic biology to treatment to lifestyle risks.[8] Starting in the mid-1990s, the emphasis in clinical cancer research shifted toward therapies derived from biotechnology research, such as gene therapy.

The concept that the immune system can recognize and destroy neoplastic cells was originally embodied in the cancer immunosurveillance hypothesis proposed by Burnet in 1957 and Thomas in 1982.[9] Unfortunately, this hypothesis was abandoned presumably because of the absence of strong experimental evidence supporting the concept then.

New data appeared in the 1990s, however, clearly showing the existence of cancer immunosurveillance and also indicating that it may function as a component of a more general process of cancer immunoediting, which is responsible for both eliminating tumors by promoting the body's protection against neoplasia and for facilitating tumor escape from immune destruction. For example, specific non-cancer cells, such as suppressor cells that expand during neoplasia, inflammation and infection and suppress immune responses, have been shown to promote cancer metastasis.

A 1994 *Time* magazine's cover announced, in bold red letters, "Hope in the War Against Cancer," surmising that "a turning point" may have been reached. In 2001, its cover asked if the blood cancer drug Gleevec "is the breakthrough we've been waiting for."

In the early 2000s as the Cancer Genome Project stated in a 2004 review article, "a central aim of cancer research has been to identify the mutated oncogenes that are causally implicated in oncogenesis (neoplasia). Cancer research ranges from epidemiology and molecular bioscience to clinical trials to evaluate and compare the various cancer treatments. These treatments include surgery, radiation therapy, chemotherapy, hormone therapy, immunotherapy and combined treatment modalities such as chemo-radiotherapy."[10]

The mission of the American Association for Cancer Research (AACR) is to prevent and cure cancer through research, education, communication and collaboration. Through its programs and services, the AACR said it "fosters research in cancer and related biomedical science; accelerates the dissemination of new research findings among scientists and others dedicated to the conquest of cancer; promotes science education and training; and advances the understanding of cancer etiology, prevention, diagnosis and treatment throughout the world. Cancer is not a single disease, but more than 200. In the U. S. and around the world, men and women in laboratories and clinics, universities, medical centers, government and industry are working not only to overcome this affliction that claims half a million American lives each year, but also to prevent it." The AACR has more than 34,000 members.

Some oncologists, including Guy Faguet, were seeing that the "cell-kill paradigm" of chemotherapy had reached its limits. The field could not go farther without understanding the underlying cellular and genetic disease mechanisms. Cancer science and cancer therapy had to be brought together. Later in 2008, Dr. Faguet exposed the "40-year stagnation in the treatment of advanced-stage cancer and its root causes and urged abandoning the failed chemotherapy model that is based on the delusion that high doses of cell-toxic agents can selectively kill cancer cells while sparing their normal counterparts."[11]

Popularizing Cancer

Mukherjee notes that the contemporary popular story of cancer started in 1940 with Albert and Mary Lasker who founded a philanthropic cause to harness the tremendous power of medical research to cure diseases. By the time Albert died of colon cancer in 1952, Mary Lasker and her supporters (by then known as the Laskerites) had begun to develop a target and a strategy: cancer was the enemy, and Washington, DC, was the battlefield. "You were probably the first person to realize that the War against Cancer has to be fought first on the floor of Congress," the breast-cancer activist Rose Kushner later wrote to Lasker, and the military language stuck. This was to be a colossal fight, needing huge amounts of money and engaging the enemy through overwhelming force.

The Laskerites needed a researcher to give the campaign credibility and to identify strategic targets. When Lasker met the cancer researcher Sidney Farber in Washington in the late 1940s, it was, Mukherjee wrote, "like the meeting of two stranded travelers, each carrying one-half of a map." In 1947, working at Boston's Children's Hospital, Farber had striking success in treating child leukemia patients with chemicals known as folic-acid antagonists. Cancers were understood to be malignant neoplasms caused by uncontrollably dividing cells. Farber was looking for substances that could target and check that division. There had been recent signs that the chemical-warfare agent nitrogen mustard could do this with non-Hodgkin's lymphoma, and it seemed that anti-foliates could be effective with certain cancers of the blood. Farber's success was limited, but, given the state of cancer therapy then, it was stunning. He was getting significant remissions through drugs. This was the origin of modern chemotherapy.

Lasker found her field commander in Farber. She capitalized on his expertise, and she eventually lifted his sights from voluntary fund-raising to political action. Working together for two decades, the pair learned how to mobilize, organize and focus scientific and technological assets. By 1970, as the Vietnam War ate away at the nation's soul and resources, Richard Nixon came to think that a War on Cancer could be much more popular than that a real war and more likely to end in an unambiguous victory. It could be another Manhattan or Apollo Project.

In his 1971 State of the Union speech, President Nixon proposed "an intensive campaign to find a cure for cancer" in what was supposed to be a "moonshot" effort to cure the disease. On December 23, 1971, he launched the War on Cancer by signing the National Cancer Act, tapping vast federal resources specifically targeted at cancer research and control. Cancer was set apart from other dread diseases; it had a special political base and a special scientific and clinical agenda. The modern cancer world came into being thanks to a new configuration of federal politics, popular activism, finance, corporate activity and science. Lasker's realization that the cure for a disease could proceed through political action changed the rules of the game.

Sidney Farber, for one, embraced the notion of the War on Cancer as a means of insisting on pressing the priority of treatment by any means. Aspirin, after all, had relieved headaches long before anyone understood how it did so. Perhaps cancer could be cured without physicians being able to specify the mechanisms of curative actions. Absent secure knowledge of fundamental mechanisms, cancer medicine in the sixties and seventies deployed the "full armamentarium of cytotoxic drugs," Mukherjee writes, "driving the body to the edge of death to rid it of its malignant innards." For practical purposes, cancer therapy and cancer science then belonged to virtually separate worlds.

The Emergence of Contemporary Cancer Treatment

Three ways to treat cancer emerged: you can cut it out surgically; you can burn it up with radiation; and you can poison it by filling the body with toxic chemicals that knock out cancer cells without enough damage to normal cells to kill the patient.

For the surgical approach, radical mastectomies didn't work; the survival rate depended not on the width of the surgical margin but on the cancer's metastatic reach before surgery. If you needed to take out a lot of tissue, the cancer had probably already spread through the system. But an ingrained surgical culture saw success as the absence of "local recurrence." Mukherjee reckons that surgeons looked the facts in the face and then looked away.

In chemotherapy, too, the lines between cruelty and cure have not always been obvious nor have consciences always been untroubled. Experience with chemotherapy led to the conviction that the ingenious adaptability of each cancer cell had to be combatted by using varied "cocktails" of chemical toxins, by continuing chemotherapy long after signs of remission and by delivering doses that might cause excruciating pain to patients and also constitute a danger to their lives.

Oncologists have faced the dilemma of whether their chief responsibility is to minimize an individual patient's suffering or to further the search for an eventual cure. When risks to a given patient may mean benefits to future sufferers, the boundary between care and experimentation can blur. Describing experimental chemotherapy regimens of the early sixties, Mukherjee recounts the controversial decisions made to concoct terrifyingly toxic cocktails for child leukemia patients, while the physicians in charge did what pathetically little they could to make the kids more comfortable. Years afterward, and with the clearer conscience of substantial success, one oncologist recognized the dangers of what they had done: "We could have killed all of those kids."

The oncologist's predicament is the precarious balance between best-practice care and the crying need to improve current practice. In the nineteen eighties, AIDS patients started to insist on being "guinea pigs", and terminal-cancer sufferers less deliberately soon followed their lead. In the current world of end-stage cancer, care and experiment often can be much the same thing.

According to American Society of Clinical Oncology, two of three people live at least five years after a cancer diagnosis now, up from roughly one of two in the 1970s.[12] About 68% of today's cancer survivors were diagnosed with cancer five or more years ago. Approximately 15% of all cancer survivors were diagnosed 20 or more years ago. More than half of cancer survivors are sixty-five or older, and 5% are younger than forty. These statistics mean that 32% of cancer victims die within 5 years of the initial diagnosis with a total of 85% dying within 20 years.

All of this must be taken in the context of the rising death toll from cancer over the years. According to the U. S. National Center for Health Statistics, from 1900 to 2005 the death rate from cancer increased by 300% whereas the death rate from cardiovascular diseases declined by 17%. According to the Surveillance, Epidemiology and End Results program of the National Cancer Institute, in 2012 there were an estimated 1,638,910 newly diagnosed persons with cancer in the United States, and 577,190 died from cancer.

We need to be reminded that diseases like tuberculosis dropped from 194 to .2/100,000 population) and influenza/pneumonia dropped from 202 to 21/100,000 and have disappeared from sight as causes of death.

As oncologists and biomedical scientists seek ever more effective interventions, why aren't we winning this decades-old War on Cancer?

The Failing War on Cancer

Oncologist Guy Faguet credits the National Cancer Institute with "the nation's advances in molecular biology and the genetics of cancer."[13] He also criticizes the agency for "three decades of stagnation in cancer treatment." He concludes that treatment progress has been slow not because of the methods of clinical trial evaluation but because of continued reliance on drugs "with no relevance to the cancerous process."

Another source of failure, Faguet says, has been the preoccupation of the National Cancer Institute with the flawed cell-kill hypothesis that undergirds chemotherapy. Chemotherapy has depended on the anti-cancer activity of "non-specific and inherently inefficacious" toxic drugs and has reached "a low efficacy plateau" that cannot be breached by dose escalation, combining drugs, timing administration or other manipulations. Faguet argues for "a fundamental paradigm shift" toward cancer control based on prevention, early diagnosis and, when these fail, "controlling the aberrant molecular genetic pathways underlying the development, growth and dissemination of cancer."

Clifton Leaf expressed deep concern about the "paltry victories" against cancer in his book *The Truth in Small Doses: Why We Are Losing the War against Cancer*.[14] He cited a 1959 pamphlet that told doctors to trickle out information to cancer-stricken patients, since most of them "couldn't stand" to know the truth: the disease would kill them, and there was little that could be done about it.

Leaf's all-consuming effort to put his finger on the fundamental issues preventing progress in the treatment of cancer resulted in his award-winning 2004 article, *Why We're Losing the War on Cancer* in *Fortune* magazine.[15] He interviewed dozens of researchers, physicians and epidemiologists at leading cancer hospitals around the country; pharmacologists, biologists and geneticists at drug companies and research centers; officials at the FDA, NCI and NIH; and fundraisers, activists and patients. Yet virtually all these experts offered testimony that Leaf found, when taken together, described a dysfunctional "cancer culture"—a group think that pushes tens of thousands of physicians and scientists toward the goal of finding the tiniest improvements in treatment rather than genuine breakthroughs, that fosters isolated (and redundant) enquiries instead of cooperation and that rewards academic achievement and publications over all else.

Leaf's overall conclusion is that progress has been so slow because: 1) cancer is a brutally complex problem; 2) terrible models—the mouse models researchers use to study cancer do not accurately represent the real disease; 3) research grants incentivize researchers to focus on narrow topics and 4) a shortage of good, creative ideas with a narrow group-think mentality. Leaf is critical of what he sees as a piecemeal effort that has been captured—because of flaws in the original legislation—by individual researchers pursuing individual agendas rather than being the goal-directed, coordinated moon-shot that was envisioned back in the 1970s. At the same time, those agendas have become more and more conservative in order to appeal to risk-averse review committees that dole out the dollars. Radical thinking and serendipity have been squeezed out.

Today, blinded by the promises of targeted therapies, Leaf concludes that we have neglected a basic truth: "the 'cancer problem' is, in reality, as formidable a challenge as ever." Still, the April 2013 issue of *Time* announced "How to Cure Cancer" as roughly one hundred and forty thousand Americans died from the disease during the next three months.

Leaf argues we should be closer to an all-out cure considering our investment in the effort. The National Cancer Institute receives roughly five billion dollars per year from the federal government. If both public and private investments are to be accounted for, Leaf estimates the United States spends about sixteen billion dollars a year on cancer research. Nor is there a lack of political will to eradicate cancer, as there is to reducing carbon emissions. Leaf calls it a "bipartisan disease" that a Republican from Alabama would want defeated as much as a Democrat from Illinois. President Barack Obama said in 2009 that he would "launch a new effort to conquer a disease that has touched the life of nearly every American, including me, by seeking a cure for cancer in our time."[16]

In Leaf's telling, oncology is a hidebound field averse to risk, a culture that "has grown progressively less hospitable to new voices and ideas over the past four decades." He yearns for the likes of Sidney Farber, the unorthodox pathologist who invented chemotherapy in the late nineteen forties at Boston Children's Hospital by injecting children stricken with acute lymphoblastic leukemia (A.L.L.) with aminopterin, which prevents cancer cells from replicating. A hero in Siddhartha Mukherjee's *The Emperor of All Maladies*, Farber is largely responsible for the fact that childhood A.L.L. is a manageable disease today. But his methods broke tradition: he disobeyed superiors and conducted his own trial-and-error studies.

What made Farber an iconoclast is that he wanted to cure cancer even more than he wanted to understand it. As he would come to argue, "The three hundred and twenty-five thousand patients with cancer who are going to die this year cannot wait; nor is it necessary, in order to make great progress in the cure for cancer, for us to have the full solution of all the problems of basic research...the history of Medicine is replete with examples of cures obtained years, decades and even centuries before the mechanism of action was understood for these cures."

Leaf also points out an even more serious deficiency in

chemoprevention: biomarkers that would accurately signal neoplasia in its earliest stages have not been found. Leaf's description of "the failed biomarker hunt" explains why oncologists today are left with no choice but to wait until cancer cells develop.

The desire for an accelerated approach to cancer has antecedents in the AIDS activism of the nineteen-eighties. As Mukherjee describes it, AIDS organizations like ACT UP "made the FDA out to be a woolly bureaucratic grandfather—exacting but maddeningly slow." That had some repercussions in cancer medicine, where patients also demanded quicker access to potentially life-saving therapies. Especially in vogue by the early nineties was "megadose chemotherapy" for breast cancer, complemented by a bone marrow transplant. (The original marrow would have been destroyed by the high toxicity of the purported cure.) Yet Mukherjee notes that by early 2000, the procedure was found to have been supported by fictional studies. One of its main proponents, a South African oncologist named Werner Bezwoda, had charmed his fellow practitioners with astounding results that masked the true, fatal dangers of this excessive approach.[17] Mukherjee calls Bezwoda's influential drug trials "a fraud, an invention, a sham," yet Bezwoda was hardly the lone cheerleader for megadose chemotherapy. Any urge to hasten the War on Cancer—however justified that urge may be—must grapple with the risk of promising anecdotes curdling into hideous truths.

In the "cancer culture" Leaf describes, at each step along the way from basic science to the clinic investigators rely on models that are consistently unreliable at predicting success—to the point where hundreds of cancer drugs are thrust into the pipeline, and many are approved by the FDA, even though their proven "activity" has little benefit in treating cancer.

"It's like a Greek tragedy," Leaf was told by Andy Grove, the chairman of Intel and a prostate-cancer survivor, who for years has tried to shake this cultural mind set as a member of several cancer advisory groups. "Everybody plays his individual part to perfection, everybody does what's right by his own life, and the total just doesn't work."

Cancer is a challenge because it has a truly uncanny ability to change its identity. "The hallmark of a cancer cell is its genetic instability," said

Isaiah Fidler, professor and chair of the department of cancer biology at the M.D. Anderson Cancer Center. The cell's DNA is not fixed the way a normal cell's is. A normal cell passes on pristine copies of its three-billion-letter code to every next-generation cell. But when a cancer cell divides, it passes along to its offspring an altered copy of its DNA instructions—and even the slightest change can have gigantic effects on cell behavior. The consequence is that while cancer is thought to begin with a single cell that has mutated, the tumors eventually formed are made up of countless cellular cousins with a variety of quirky traits living side by side. "That heterogeneity of tumors is the major, major obstacle to easy therapy," Fidler said to Leaf.

Modern cancer care is big business, and cancer drugs are envisaged as the current and future cash cows of pharmaceutical companies. The expense of developing cancer drugs, and their cost to patients and insurers, would clearly be worth it if the drugs promised cures or even deep remissions, but the vast majority of new drugs achieve far more modest results.

The current cancer effort is utterly fragmented—so much so that it's nearly impossible to track down where the money to pay for all the research is coming from. When you add it all up, Leaf estimates that Americans have spent, through taxes, donations and private R&D close to $200 billion in inflation-adjusted dollars since 1971. What has that national investment netted so far?

Without question, the money has bought us an enormous amount of knowledge. Researchers have mapped a cell's intricate inner circuitry in extraordinary detail. In short, scientists now know nearly all the biochemical steps that a healthy cell uses to multiply, to shut down its growth and to sense internal damage and die at the right time—as well as many of the genes that encode for these processes. What's more they know how these same gene-induced mechanisms go haywire in cancer cells. Leaf cites PubMed's estimate that the cancer research community has published 1.56 million papers largely on this circuitry and its related genes in hundreds of journals over the years. Many of the findings are shared at the 100-plus international congresses, symposiums and conventions held each year.

Yet somehow, along the way, something important has been lost. The search for knowledge has become an end unto itself rather than the means to an end. And the research has become increasingly narrow, so much so that physician-scientists who want to think systemically about cancer or the body as a whole—or who might have completely new approaches— often can't get funding.

Take, for instance, the NCI's chief funding mechanism, called an RO1 grant. The grants are generous, averaging $338,000 apiece in 2003. And they have been one of the easiest sweepstakes to win: One in three applications have been accepted. But the money goes almost entirely to researchers who focus on very specific genetic or molecular mechanisms within the cancer cell or other tissues. The narrower the research niche, it sometimes seems, the greater the rewards the researcher is likely to attain. "The incentives are not aligned with the goals," Leonard Zwelling, vice president for research administration at M.D. Anderson, said to Leaf, voicing the feelings of many. "If the goal is to cure cancer, you don't incentivize people to have little publications."

Jean-Pierre Issa, a colleague of Zwelling's who studies leukemias, is equally frustrated by the cancer community's mindset. Still, he admits, the system's lure is powerful. "You get a paper where you change one gene ever so slightly and you have a drastic effect on cancer in the mouse, and that paper gets published in your best journals like *Science* or *Nature*. That makes your reputation. Then you start getting grants based on that. Open any major journal and 80% of it is mice or drosophila (fruit flies) or nematodes (worms). When do you get human studies in there?"

Indeed, the cancer community has published an extraordinary 150,855 experimental studies on mice, according to Leaf's search of the PubMed database. Guess how many of them have led to treatments for cancer? Very, very few.

Looking for fresh insights into cancer research, the National Institutes for Health in 2009 launched 12 physical science oncology centers at universities around the United States. The funders hope cancer research, which has benefited from tools made by physicists, can also benefit from physicists' unique perspective on cancer as a physical system.

Peggy Orenstein, an author and cancer survivor, said we're squandering time, money and resources.[18] When facing the helplessness of a disease, it feels good to believe we are somehow collectively "battling" it. It feels good enough, in fact, to have turned breast cancer into a big, Pepto Bismol-colored business, and to have driven unprecedented droves of women into prophylactic mastectomies.

Yet reality is far more complicated than a jaunty ribbon on a lapel or the hopeful promise of "early detection." That point is well-illustrated in Orenstein's blistering cover story for the *New York Times Magazine* on "Our Feel-Good War on Breast Cancer."[19] She knows well the nightmare of breast cancer. She was diagnosed in 1996 at the age of 35. A decade and a half later, she was diagnosed again. And that span of time represents a massive shift in our cultural relationship with breast cancer—and a surprising new concern: what she calls "the dangers of overtreatment."

As Orenstein writes, a mammogram like the one that first detected her cancer does "reduce, by a small percentage, the number of women who are told they have late-stage cancer, but it is far more likely to result in overdiagnosis and unnecessary treatment, including surgery, weeks of radiation, and potentially toxic drugs." Of particular interest to Orenstein are the 60,000 new diagnoses annually—roughly a quarter of them of ductal carcinoma in situ (DCIS). Also known as "Stage O," DCIS is not cancer, just the presence of abnormal cells that could become cancer. Complicating matters is the fact that, as Orenstein notes, "There are at least four genetically distinct breast cancers. Mammograms, it turns out, are not so great at detecting the most lethal forms of disease."

The presence of any unusual cells, of course, remains a scary red flag, and Orenstein observes that action has a more can-do appeal than wait-and-see. That's likely why the same tremendous progress we've made in detection has led—and not necessarily helpfully— to a 188 percent jump between 1998 and 2005 among women given new diagnoses of DCIS in one breast … who opted to have both breasts removed just in case and a stunning 150 percent rise among women with early-stage invasive disease.

As Orenstein told *Salon*, "We've been lulled into a false sense of security. I felt that some of the issues around mammography and DCIS—and the idea that it was being seen as a triumph of early detection instead of a casualty of it—weren't being put together in a big coherent way."

"Surviving" something that might never have grown into a severe threat makes for a happy-ending story. Having a disease that's genuinely out to kill you? Still alarmingly taboo. It's strange–for all our talk about "the cure" so little attention and research and funding actually goes to treat the people who need a cure the most.

Conclusion

Cancer always has been with us. Its care and management have differed over time, but so, too, have its identity, visibility, meanings and frequency. Because we are living longer and our environments and foods are polluted with cancer causing agents, cancer has become the leading cause of death in the world.

The experience of cancer has always been terrible, but, until modern times, its effect on our society has been light. In the past, the common fear was of dying from other causes: infectious diseases; "apoplexies"; and, most notably in the nineteenth century, "consumption". The agonizing manner of cancer death was dreaded, but that fear was not centrally situated in the public mind—as it now is.

In his 1971 State of the Union speech, President Nixon proposed "an intensive campaign to find a cure for cancer" in what was supposed to be a "moonshot" effort to cure the disease. On December 23, 1971, he launched the War on Cancer by signing the National Cancer Act.

Cancer cells present a daunting challenge because they have a truly uncanny ability to change their identities. As a result, the three traditional ways to treat cancer—surgery, radiation and chemotherapy—have not won the War on Cancer. Our scientific approach to cancer also has been handicapped by fragmentation, discontinuity and the lack of a focus on how cancer cells are produced and multiply through the process of neoplasia.

How Cancer Cells Form and Multiply

The process of neoplasia is described as well as how the immune system normally holds this process in check and also can fail to do so thereby permitting cancer cells to grow and spread.

Uncommon in early life, cancer appears predominantly during later life. It's almost as if evolution protected us during our childbearing years and abandoned us after we no longer had procreative value.

Although aging in itself is an obvious risk factor for cancer, it's also clear that prolonged exposure to toxins in the environment can cause cancer. It appears that cancer is connected with our inflammatory response to injury to cells. If you smoke, you damage your lung cells...and lung cancer arises. If you drink excessively, you damage your liver cells...and liver cancer occurs. If you have a bone fracture...bone cancer may appear. As you age, there is a greater likelihood of normal cell processes faltering and breaking down. When cancer cells form, it's like your body is trying to respond to damaged cells but can't control the repair process.

Your body's natural defenses create an inhospitable environment for cancer growth. It's clear that a cancer cell or a tumor is not a self-contained system and requires a hospitable environment in which to grow. It's a cell or tumor that is interacting abnormally with a variety of systems in its immediate environment—its *microenvironment*—that ordinarily support the natural death of your cells by what is called *apoptosis*. (This word is derived from ancient Greek for the falling away of petals from a flower or leaves from a tree.) The microenvironment is the terrain that largely determines whether cancer cells will grow or not. These microenvironmental factors include the propensity for inflammation, the suppression of immune cells and the ability to form blood vessels to feed a growing tumor (angiogenesis). The reasons why a cell becomes a cancer cell lie within the cell and its microenvironment.

As you read this, millions of your cells are dying. Most of them are either superfluous or potentially harmful, so you're better off without them. In fact, your health depends on the normal death of your cells—apoptosis.

Apoptosis

Apoptosis, or programmed cell death, is a naturally occurring process in your body. Except for brain, heart and bone cells, most cells in your body have a life span of less than 10 years. For example, your colon cells last about four days, epidermal cells two weeks, red blood cells four months, white blood cells a year and muscle cells fifteen years.

In apoptosis, a cell's genes trigger a process that allows it to "commit suicide." The cell shrinks and pulls away from its neighbors. Then, the surface of the cell appears to boil with fragments breaking away. The DNA in the nucleus condenses and breaks into fragments followed by breakdown of the nucleus. Next the entire cell disintegrates into smaller fragments that are enclosed in membranes so as not to harm neighboring cells. A cellular cleanup crew (the immune system) rapidly mops up the cell's remains without causing an inflammatory reaction.

Your cells are equipped with the instructions and instruments necessary for their own self-destruction. They keep these tools tucked away, like a set of sheathed knives, until some signal—either from within or outside the cell—triggers their release. This initiates a cascade of carefully coordinated events that culminate in the efficient, pain-free excision of your unneeded cells.

How do your cells know when to die? It turns out that each cell has 92 internal clocks—one at each end of its 46 chromosomes. Before a cell divides, it copies its chromosomes so that each offspring cell will get a complete set. Telomeres protect each end of a chromosome from deterioration or from fusion with neighboring chromosome. With each cell division, its telomeres are shortened slightly. Once a cell's telomeres shrink to a critical minimum size, the cell takes notice and stops dividing and shows the signs of aging familiar to all of us.

After cells divide about 50 times, they quit the hard work of dividing and enter a phase in which they no longer behave as they did previously. This may be why most cancers occur in later life. Regardless of age cancer cells result from the process of neoplasia.

Neoplasia

Hyperplasia is a normal physiological response to demand placed on a tissue to produce more cells. When their division becomes poorly regulated, cells lose some of their characteristics and/or functions. The tissue they comprise becomes disordered in appearance, often with an increase in the numbers of immature cells and greater variability between cells. This appearance is called dysplasia, which may or may not be a stage on the way to neoplasia.

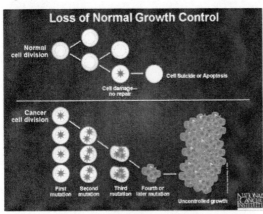

Neoplasia
(From National Cancer Institute
Understanding Cancer Series: Cancer)

Neoplasia is an abnormal process in our bodies in which our cells do not die through apoptosis after a normal life span but continue to live and reproduce without being detected and eliminated by our immune systems. Our bodies consist of trillions of cells that live in harmony unless certain cells withdraw from cooperating with the others through the process of neoplasia and become cancer cells that are jobless, homeless and living off other cells.

Neoplasia is the multiplication of a cell by abnormally dividing and forming new cells. The multiplication of neoplastic cells exceeds, and is not coordinated with, that of the normal cells around them. That growth persists even after the stimulus that caused it stops. These aberrant cells are not destroyed by the immune system and join to form benign or malignant (cancer) tumors or remain independent as blood cancer cells. So cancer cells are the products of neoplasia. Cancer is not a disease in itself. It's a product (in medical terms a physical sign) of the disease neoplasia.

When the normal cycles of life and death of your body's cells go awry, aberrant cells undergo neoplasia and become benign or malignant tumors...cancer. Although the forms of cancer cells vary widely, the underlying disease—neoplasia—is the same throughout the body. Neoplasia occurs when your body's immune system fails to recognize and destroy aberrant cells for a variety of reasons.

At least one in three persons will receive the diagnosis of cancer. The immune systems of those of us who have not yet received the diagnosis have been destroying potential cancer cells up until now...as far as we know.

The Process of Neoplasia

A variety of factors cause cells to escape regulation by normal body processes. First of all, since cells are constantly dividing and are copying their own DNA, random errors inevitably arise with an increasing tendency to do so the longer you live. Some DNA copying errors are inevitable due to the sheer volume of replication that occurs every day, and aging cells tend to make more errors in DNA replication than younger cells. So there's an inherent tradeoff in cell division: it allows you to grow to maturity and keeps you healthy, but it's also the source of potentially damaging DNA mutations.[1] Fortunately, almost all of these errors are corrected by your extremely efficient DNA repair systems.

DNA Damage

You have a signaling pathway, called the DNA damage detection response, to protect you against insults to your DNA. Normal DNA is like a relatively straight, stiff piece of rubber. It becomes possible to bend the DNA in places where there are defects. The DNA damage detection machinery seems to take advantage of this propensity by testing DNA to determine whether it can be bent easily. When it can, repair is initiated.

Your DNA damage detection response activates DNA repair functions, such that cells with modest damage are likely to survive. However, cells with more severe damage are induced to undergo apoptosis. The DNA damage detection response is activated very early during neoplasia so that it functions as a barrier to the progression of neoplasia. A 2006 study demonstrated that, when the DNA damage detection response finds a cell with unmanageable DNA damage, it alerts the immune system which activates Natural Killer T cells that destroy the cell.[2] These findings have important implications for designing cancer therapies and for drug development.

If your DNA repair system does not do its job, most aberrant cells die anyway because they are abnormal enough for the body's immune system to destroy them. However, if factors promoting neoplasia exist, misbehaving cells give rise to cancer cells that continue to multiply.

In addition to elements in an aberrant cell's microenvironment that provide cover for neoplasia, there are two principal reasons why the immune system fails to hold neoplasia in check. One is that cells innately evade the immune system because of a genetic predisposition, or they are influenced by environmental toxins to do so. These possibilities are the basis for genomic research. The second reason is that the immune system has a genetic predisposition to breakdown or is induced to malfunction by external or internal toxins or just by the aging process itself. These possibilities are the basis for immunological research.

Your body cells are constantly exposed to DNA damage from your external environment in the form of radiation, chemicals and viral infections. Metabolic processes within your cells also can generate free radicals that threaten the integrity of your cells including their DNA (described in detail in Chapter Ten). DNA damage promotes neoplasia.

Cancer cells can develop in anyone through the process of neoplasia, although there may be predispositions in some persons to do so. Susceptibility to cancers resulting from environmental exposure may be inherited if a parent is exposed to a carcinogen that causes egg or sperm cell genetic changes that subsequently are passed on to a child.

The basic question, then, is how does your immune system keep you free of cancer cells most of the time? The answer is clear-cut. Normally your immune system recognizes and eliminates neoplastic cells because they do not fit a pattern that is recognized as a normal part of the body. So why does your immune system fail to recognize cells that grow out of control and become cancer?

In a landmark review, Douglas Hanahan and Robert Weinberg described seven alterations in cell physiology that underlie cancer cell growth through neoplasia.[3]

1) abnormal "go" signals,
2) insensitivity to "stop" signals,
3) evasion of normal programmed cell death (apoptosis),
4) limitless replicative potential,
5) sustained growth of its own blood supply,
6) invasion and metastasis and
7) reprogramming of energy metabolism

Your body carefully controls how and when your cells divide and multiply by using molecular "stop" and "go" signals.[4] For example, injured cells at the site of a wound send "go" signals to the surrounding skin cells, which respond by dividing and multiplying to seal the wound with a scar through the process of inflammation. Conversely, "stop" signals are generated when a cell finds itself in in a nutrient-poor environment. Sometimes "go" signals are produced when they shouldn't be, or "stop" signals aren't sent or heeded. Both scenarios can result in uncontrolled cell division and consequent cancer cells as the wound repairing inflammatory process goes awry. This has led to characterizing cancer as "wounds that never heal."[5]

Fortunately, it takes more than one mistaken "stop" or "go" signal for a cell to become cancer. Because your body is good at protecting your essential systems, it usually requires at least a one-two punch for healthy cells to turn malignant. The punches come in the form of a sequence of errors—mutations—in damaged DNA that result in the production of aberrant cells. Inflammation caused by sunlight, radiation, toxins in cigarette smoke and air and water pollution and some viruses and parasites can cause such mutations. A few people also can inherit mutations from their parents, which explains why some families have higher rates of certain cancers; the first punch is delivered at conception. Subsequent gene mutations then can push cells down the path toward becoming cancer.

Cancer Cells Revert to Primitive State

Under normal circumstances chromosomes are only copied once before a cell divides, otherwise this can lead to genetic diseases and cancer. In the process of neoplasia aberrant cells no longer regulate copying of their genes because of mutations in the genes that control cell reproduction. It's as if cancer cells revert back to a more primitive state that does not have these forms of control, like in embryonic tissues. Aggressive cancer cells grow faster than ordinary cells and can quickly spread throughout your body. In an evolutionary sense, cancer cells are much better prepared for survival than normal cells. They are selfishly growing rapidly and thriving at the expense of surrounding cells and your body..."the survival of the fittest". Like embryonic cells, they can change into different forms.

Cancer cells even can change their shapes and travel through tissues.[6] They can disguise themselves so that they can deceive and bypass your immune system, including building skins that shield tumors they form from your immune system and from drugs. They can be enabled by elements in the micro-environment that suppress your immune system and that provide cover for neoplasia. In addition, defects in your immune system can make it blind to neoplasia and its resulting cancer cells.

Environmental Toxins

Increasing scientific evidence suggests that cancer is driven by oxidative stress and inflammation attributable to environmental factors that either drive genetic mutations or modify the expression of key regulatory genes.[7] According to the U.S. Department of Health and Human Services, over 70,000 manufactured chemicals are being sold today. Over 350 of them have been identified as carcinogenic in humans…as stimulating neoplasia. The true number is higher since the program has not been able to conduct screenings on the majority of chemicals on the market. A variety of chemical carcinogens as diverse as benzene, cigarette smoke, nitrates and nitrites may initiate and/or promote the process of neoplasia. Radiation—either as low level long-term environmental gamma rays or as higher dose therapeutic radiation—also can produce DNA damage and genetic mutations in cells. These and many more suspected carcinogens are correlated with the rise and fall of cancer rates over the years, but priority has not been given to research on how these toxins affect the immune system. For example, we do not know how the over 32 known carcinogenic chemicals in tobacco smoke affect the immune system. Instead, the dominant focus has been on the genes of cancer cells rather than on the genes of immune system cells.

Infection Related Factors in Neoplasia

2011 marked the centenary of Francis Peyton Rous's landmark experiments on an avian cancer virus. Examples of microbes that have been found to cause 15–20% of human cancers worldwide are the bacterium *Heliobactor pylori* (stomach cancer); viruses, such as the human papillomavirus (cervical and oropharyngeal cancers), hepatitis B and C (liver cancer), and the Epstein-Barr virus (nasopharyngeal cancer and some lymphomas); and the parasite *Clonorchis sinensis* (gall bladder cancer).[8] This diverse group of microbes reveals connections between the way the immune system responds to both infections and cancer.

Viruses establish long-term persistent infections in humans that have cancer as an accidental side effect of viral replication strategies. They usually interact with other environmental factors in order to induce neoplasia. Many years may pass between initial infection and tumor appearance. Most infected individuals do not develop cancer, so persons with deficient immune systems are at elevated risk for viral-associated cancers.

For these cancers, infection is only one component in the ultimate causes of their neoplasia. But the importance of virally influenced cancers has not been fully appreciated leading to overlooked opportunities in cancer control.

Genetic Factors in Neoplasia

The Cancer Genome Atlas has analyzed over 100,000 cancer cases across 27 tumor types. One of the findings is that cancer tumors from the same type of tissue often have different genetic traits, while those from different tissues frequently are similar.[9]

James Watson, co-discoverer of the structure of DNA in 1953 with Francis Crick, was filled with optimism in the summer of 2009 about the genetic theory of cancer.[10] Oncogenes—mutations of normal genes that can be inherited or caused by exposure to toxic substances in the environment—were thought to be directly responsible for cells becoming cancer cells. In the winter of 2012, he was equally filled with scathing pessimism when the random nature of mutations in cancer cells caught him and everybody by surprise.

It seemed to Watson as though cancer had dangled a carrot in front of him, only to jerk it back as he cautiously reached out with hope. He declared, "the 'curing' of many cancers seems now to many seasoned scientists an even more daunting objective than when the War on Cancer was started by President Nixon in December 1971. The biggest obstacle today to moving forward effectively towards a true war against cancer may, in fact, come from the inherently conservative nature of today's cancer research establishments." Watson concluded that defective metabolism underlies cancer. He called it the "Achilles Heel" of the cancer cell that should be the focus of research.

Bert Vogelstein, a cancer researcher at Johns Hopkins University, finally concluded that enough data was compiled to conclusively determine that the idea of a tidy series of sequential mutations as the cause of cancer should be scrapped.[11] In its place, Vogelstein holds that rather than a defined set of specific mutations being the cause of a given cancer, cancer is a cellular systems disease. A given system might have 20 or so genes required to operate—so the theory goes. If any single one of the genes is rendered dysfunctional by a mutation, then the whole system becomes non-operational, marching the cell one step closer to neoplasia and becoming a cancer cell.

The flaw in the genetic theory is that oncogene mutations, although just a side effect of the true origin of cancer, were easily mistaken as the cause—sending researchers on a multi-billion dollar and multi-decade misdirected chase and creating excessive public worry. An example is the BRAC1 genetic mutation in cancer of the ovary and breast, which recently caught the public's attention as the mutation responsible for Angelina Jolie's decision to undergo a double mastectomy. Inheriting a faulty BRAC1 gene does jump the risk of acquiring breast cancer in a women's lifetime to 60% from 12%. However, Stanford University Cancer Institute's Diana Zuckerman argues that "Since being overweight and smoking increase the risk and exercising and breastfeeding lower the risk, Ms. Jolie's risk of breast cancer, even with the BRCA1 gene, could be considerably lower. If any woman with BRCA1 gets breast cancer in the future, the treatments available would be even more effective than they are today."[12]

An elegant series of nucleus transfer experiments reveal the true nature of cancer. They consist of transferring the nucleus of a cancer cell into a healthy cell that has had its nucleus removed. The newly created hybrid cell has the genetic material (DNA) of a cancer cell, with all of its defects, but still has the healthy mitochondria of a normal cell. Intuitively, if the origin of cancer is indeed mutations to nuclear DNA, the newly created hybrid cells that now have all of the mutations should be cancer cells. But they are not. Experiments like these provide strong evidence that ultimately nuclear DNA mutations are not in the driver's seat with respect to the origin of cancer; the mitochondria are.[13]

Metabolic Factors in Neoplasia

Long before the cause of cancer was thought to be genetic it was thought to be metabolic. Metabolism is a general word describing all of the chemical reactions a cell undergoes to generate energy for its work and to multiply. It is the primary job of your mitochondria.

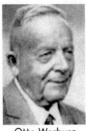
Otto Warburg

Otto Warburg, a chemist and physician, postulated in 1924 that the primary cause of cancer is the replacement of oxygen metabolism in normal body cells by the fermentation of sugar.[14] He was nominated an unprecedented three times for the Nobel Prize and single handedly advanced human physiology by leaps and bounds in the early twentieth century. Since Warburg was a Jew in Nazi Germany, he was unable to accept a second Nobel Prize Award in 1944. Nevertheless, he was not persecuted, because Hitler was afraid of cancer, and Warburg was the world's foremost expert then.

In 1952, Ernst Krebs, Jr., a biochemist in San Francisco, advanced the theory that cancer, like scurvy and pellagra, is not caused by some kind of mysterious bacteria, virus or toxin but is a deficiency disease aggravated by the lack of essential nutritional elements in modern diets.[15] However, his metabolic theory was put aside when the emphasis was placed on the DNA mutations of cancer cells.

Your normal cells have two ways to convert the glucose generated from the food you eat into your body's primary energy source—adenosine 5'-triphosphate (ATP). The first is by glycolysis in the cytoplasm of your cells (called "fermentation"). The second, and more important way, is the tricarboxylic (Krebs-TCA) cycle and oxidative phosphorylation (OxPhos) in your cells' mitochondria. This is called a cell's "respiration" because it uses the oxygen in the air you breathe to produce ATP. In addition the amino acid glutamine derived from the protein you eat is converted into alpha-ketoglutarate through the mitochondrial Krebs-TCA-OxPhos process resulting in ATP formation. All normal cells require a relatively constant level of ATP to function well and derive the majority of it from "respiration" in their mitochondria and only a small amount from "fermentation" in their cytoplasm.

The "Warburg effect" refers to the way cancer cells predominantly produce energy by a high rate of "fermentation" in their cytoplasm outside of their mitochondria. "Fermentation" produces lactic acid and a little ATP in contrast with the highly efficient "respiration" that produces ATP in your normal cells. Rapidly growing malignant cells typically have "fermentation" rates up to 200 times higher than those of normal cells. "Fermentation" is an inefficient way to generate ATP, so cancer cells must consume extremely large amounts of glucose and glutamine to survive. In the process, high levels of lactic acid are produced that may contribute to the invasion of surrounding tissues and metastasis.

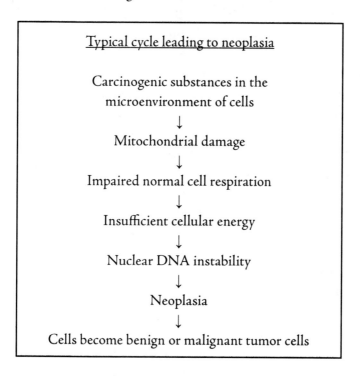

Mitochondria have their own DNA. Carcinogenic substances in the microenvironment of cells, such as environmental toxins, viruses and chronic inflammation, stimulate the production of reactive oxygen species (ROS)—also called free radicals—that are the waste byproduct of oxygen metabolism. When ROS reach too high levels in normal cells, they damage the mitochondrial DNA so that the mitochondria become abnormal structurally and functionally. This impairs the "respiration" of normal cells, which leads to mitochondrial damage, insufficient energy, nuclear DNA instability and uncontrolled cell proliferation. This begins the process of neoplasia.

Current knowledge about what is called epigenetic signaling (signaling from elements outside of the nuclear DNA) reveals that unlike the fixed DNA genetic code in a cell's nucleus, metabolic epigenetic drivers are fluid and transient forces that influence the expression of DNA. Dr. Thomas Seyfried and others now propose that chronic and persistent damage to the mitochondria in cells ultimately triggers an epigenetic signal from the mitochondria to the nuclear DNA, altering the expression of a plethora of cancer causing genes...a classic epigenetic system.[16] The BRAC1 genetic mutation previously mentioned is involved in impeding mitochondrial function, including the growth of new mitochondria. Therefore, an inherited mutation to BRAC1 would show up in reduced mitochondrial capacity—the metabolic origin of cancer.

Gleevec, the successful cancer targeted drug for the treatment of chronic myelogenous leukemia, is often cited as proof of the principle that targeting drugs on oncogenes is the right strategy. A closer look reveals that Gleevec exerts its anti-cancer effect by altering a defective metabolism pathway. Seyfried noted, "Gleevec simply highjacks a random mutation that serendipitously down-regulates an oncogenic pathway turned-on by damaged mitochondria."

If there is a modern-day incarnation of Otto Warburg, he is Dr. Peter Pedersen of John Hopkins school of Medicine in Baltimore. If the Warburg theory of cancer was a raging fire in the early 20th century, then it dimmed to a single ember by the middle of the century...an ember that Dr. Pedersen nurtured and kept alive.[17] Pedersen said, "I've watched interest in the metabolism of cancer go down to zero in the 1970's, but now interest is returning. There were times in my early career when I felt almost alone in considering energy metabolism as important to the cancer problem. I even remember one of my colleagues, an expert in DNA technology, dumping Lehninger's "Warburg Flasks" in the trash as relics of a bygone era in cancer research."

Following in the footsteps of Warburg and caught in the midst of an unpleasant anti-Warburg, anti-metabolic era, Pedersen and his collaborators quietly began to identify the key molecular events involved in the "Warburg effect" that causes the excessive consumption of glucose by cancer cells. The mitochondria of cancer cells are involved through glycolysis in providing the necessary energy to fuel their rapid growth. Also, the mitochondria hold the secrets to the immortality of cancer cells and their propensity to spread (metastasize) from their original site of origin to other parts of the body.[18]

The most common metabolic hallmark of cancer tumors is their propensity to ferment glucose to lactic acid at a high rate even in the presence of oxygen ("Warburg effect"). More than three decades ago Pedersen's laboratory showed that the pivotal player is mitochondrial-bound hexokinase (HK-2), which is a marker of cancer now used in clinics worldwide in one of the most common imaging systems for detecting cancer—positron emission tomography (PET scans).[19] By stationing itself on the outer mitochondrial membrane, HK-2 helps cancer cells grow and escape inhibition.

With the re-emergence and acceptance of the "Warburg effect" as a prominent characteristic of most cancers, a number of laboratories are now focusing on "metabolic targeting" as a therapeutic strategy. One promising anti-cancer agent is 3-bromopyruvate (3BP) discovered as such by Dr. Young H. Ko while working in the Pedersen laboratory. Significantly, 3BP kills cancer cells effectively by inhibiting their energy production pathways while leaving most normal cells alone.[20]

Emotional Stress

Links between emotional stress and cancer can arise in several ways. For example, people under stress develop behaviors, such as smoking, overeating or drinking alcohol, that increase their risks for cancer. Stress also can indirectly promote cancer by weakening the immune system through releasing high levels of the hormones cortisol and epinephrine (adrenaline). Studies have shown that these hormones make breast, ovarian and prostate cancer cells resistant to destruction.[21]

Autoimmune Diseases

Normally, your immune system protects your body against infections caused by bacteria, viruses and other parasites. It recognizes when something foreign enters your body and can usually get rid of it before it causes you any harm. But if you have an autoimmune disease, your immune system can make mistakes and attack your own normal body cells.

Generally if you have an autoimmune disease you are not significantly more likely to get cancer than other people. But some studies have reported a positive association between cancer and 23 autoimmune and inflammatory diseases, such as celiac disease, inflammatory bowel disease, rheumatoid arthritis, systemic lupus erythematosus and multiple sclerosis.[22] More specifically, people who have coeliac disease have a higher risk of nonHodgkin's lymphoma, and men who have a treatment called PUVA for psoriasis can have a higher risk of penile cancer. Less frequently some autoimmune conditions develop in the course of some cancers, such as vitiligo in melanoma.

Neoplasia as an Ancient and Embryonic Response to Stress

A new theory challenges the orthodox view that cancer develops anew in each host by a series of chance mutational accidents. Paul Davies of Arizona State University and Charles Lineweaver of the Australian National University propose that cancer actually is an organized and systematic response to stress or physical challenge. It might be triggered by a random accident, they say, but thereafter it more or less predictably unfolds.[23] "We envisage cancer as the execution of an ancient program pre-loaded into the genomes of all cells," said Davies. "It is like Windows defaulting to 'safe mode' after suffering an insult of some sort." As such, he describes cancer as a throwback to an ancestral process.

Both Davies and Lineweaver are theoretical physicists and cosmologists who work in astrobiology—the search for life beyond Earth. They turned to cancer research recently, in part because one of twelve centers established by the National Cancer Institute to encourage physical scientists to tackle cancer is the Beyond Center for Fundamental Concepts in Science at Arizona State University.

Their theory predicts that as neoplasia progresses through more and more malignant stages, it will express genes that are more deeply conserved among multicellular organisms, and so are in a sense more ancient. Davies and Lineweaver are currently testing this prediction by comparing gene expression data from cancer biopsies with phylogenetic trees going back 1.6 billion years, with the help of Luis Cisneros, a researcher with ASU's Beyond Center.

But if this is the case, why hasn't evolution eliminated the ancient cancer subroutine? "Because it fulfills absolutely crucial functions during the early stages of embryo development," Davies explains. "Genes that are active in the embryo and normally dormant thereafter are found to be switched back on in cancer. These same genes are the 'ancient' ones, deep in the tree of multicellular life."

Support for this theory is found in the potential role of Human Chorionic Gonadotropin (HCG) in cancer. HCG results from the fusion of sperm and egg and is the hormone detected in a pregnancy test. Progesterone closely follows HCG and assists in embryonic stem cell proliferation and differentiation. An accidental switch of the HCG gene from OFF to ON can de-differentiate an adult cell toward becoming a cancer cell, thereby enabling the cell to mimic embryonic growth, escape attack by the immune system and enter neoplasia. HCG is a sensitive and specific marker for a number of cancer types. Based on this finding the use of Mifepristone (RU-486)—an abortion drug and emergency contraceptive—is being tested as a treatment for cancer.[24]

The link with embryonic development has been known to cancer biologists for a long time, says Davies, but the significance of this fact is rarely appreciated. Our body cells are engineered to succeed by proliferating. The genes that guide embryos to grow into fully developed bodies also may enable cancer cells to proliferate if they are activated in later life. Unlike the regulated embryo that sheds off excess and aberrant cells though apoptosis, unregulated cancer cells escape self-destruction and spin further out of control. What's more, as the embryo grows it secretes enzymes that create blood vessels through a process called angiogenesis that also is used by cancer tumors to grow their own blood supply.

Intriguingly, primary heart cancer is rare after birth, largely because heart cells do not split and multiply then.[25] The only time they divide is during fetal development when heart tumors do occur. Around the time of birth, the switch that controls whether or not heart cells divide turns off. Any tumors that existed in utero generally stop growing.

If this new theory is correct, researchers should find that the malignant stages of neoplasia re-express unregulated genes from the earliest stages of embryogenesis. Davies adds that there is already some evidence for this in several experimental studies, including recent research at Harvard University and the Albert Einstein College of Medicine in New York. "As cancer progresses through its various stages within a single organism, it should be like running the evolutionary and developmental arrows of time backward at high speed," says Davies.

This theory could provide clues to future treatment. For example, when life took the momentous step from single cells to multicellular organisms, Earth had low levels of oxygen. Sure enough, cancer reverts in part to an ancient form of metabolism called fermentation or glycolysis that is less dependent on oxygen and therefore can still thrive under normal or low oxygen conditions. For example, in one liver cancer cell line where this was carefully studied, it was found that 60% of the ATP was derived from glycolysis and the remaining 40% from mitochondrial oxidative phosphorylation.[26]

Davies and Lineweaver predict that if cancer cells are saturated with oxygen but deprived of glucose, they will become more stressed than healthy cells, slowing them down or even killing them. "It is clear that some radically new thinking is needed," Davies said. "Like aging, cancer seems to be a deeply embedded part of the life process. Also like aging, cancer generally cannot be cured but its effects can certainly be mitigated, for example, by delaying onset and extending periods of dormancy. But we will learn to do this effectively only when we better understand cancer, including its place in the great sweep of evolutionary history."[27]

Conclusion

Galen was right. Although most obvious in cancers of the blood, all cancers are diseases of the whole body, not just where the tumors appear. For this reason just removing or destroying cancer tumors doesn't remove the condition that caused them in the first place. That's why cancer often returns after conventional treatment.

The more science tells us about cancer cells the more they resemble human beings. They want to grow and multiply, as we do, but they don't know how to stop. Researchers, in their more detached moments, can't help admiring the cancer cell, the way that Sherlock Holmes admired Moriarty as an evil, but worthy, opponent.

Neoplasia is an abnormal process in our bodies in which cells do not die after a normal life span through what is called apoptosis but continue to live and reproduce without being detected and eliminated by our immune systems. So cancer cells are the products of neoplasia. Cancer is not a disease in itself. It's a product of the disease neoplasia.

The metabolic theory of neoplasia provides a simple and elegant explanation for cancer development and metastasis that is in complete harmony with empirical evidence in contrast to the genetic theory. Einstein's statement, "the simplest explanation is usually the correct one" might well apply here.

Chapter Six

Cancer Research

*The pro and cons of the way cancer research
has been conducted are presented.*

In its 2011 report *Accelerating Progress Against Cancer*, the American Society of Clinical Oncologists (ASCO) concluded that cancer research and patient care should be "vastly more targeted, more efficient and more effective."[1] The report expressed the hope that if recent advances are pursued, it is not unrealistic to imagine that over the next decade clinicians will increasingly be able to choose therapies that target the characteristics of each cancer and each patient. Cancer diagnosis will be earlier, and diagnostic tests will provide detailed information for making treatment decisions and the management of side effects.

But ASCO pointed out that this vision is possible only if we transform the way cancer research is conducted. The nation's cancer drug development and clinical research infrastructures have not kept pace with recent advances. The clinical trial system has been weakened by a labyrinth of regulatory requirements and years of underfunding. Traditional clinical trial designs and drug development models are insufficient to fully capitalize on the potential of targeted therapies. Unfortunately, drug companies have been discouraged from sharing ideas or testing promising new treatments in combination due to a lack of incentives to do so and the absence of a clear process for collaboration.

In 2014 ASCO appealed to patients, patient advocates and clinical investigators to collectively raise the bar and design clinical trials to demonstrate greater "clinically meaningful outcomes" for advanced pancreatic, lung, breast and colon cancers.[2]

ASCO's appeal reflects the fact that currently there is no consensus among researchers or research funders about the most urgent and promising priorities for diagnostic and treatment development. In addition, trial sponsors often focus on areas that are unlikely to result in major advances over existing options, while critical gaps in cancer prevention and treatment are left unaddressed.

The 2011 ASCO report stressed that improving strategies for the prevention and treatment of cancer will require teams of researchers. Academic incentives, however, reward individual research efforts over team approaches. In addition, legal, financial, patent and regulatory hurdles currently make it challenging for companies to work together to test promising combinations of treatments.

All of this is taking place in the context of problems with scientific research in general. According to *The Economist* magazine, too many of the findings that fill the academic ether are the result of shoddy experiments or poor analysis.[3] A rule of thumb among biotechnology venture-capitalists is that half of published research cannot be replicated. From 2000-2010 roughly 80,000 patients took part in clinical trials based on research that was later retracted because of mistakes or improprieties.

According to the editorial board of the prestigious journal *Nature*, no research paper can ever be considered to be the final word. The replication and corroboration of research results is key to the scientific process.[4] *Nature* has published a series of articles about the worrying extent to which research results have been found wanting.

John Ioannidis, a meta-researcher who researchs research, concluded that contradictions and initially stronger effects are not unusual in highly cited research on clinical interventions and their outcomes.[5] Controversies are most common with nonrandomized studies, but even the most highly cited randomized trials may be challenged and refuted over time. Dr. Ioannidis and Steven Goodman established the Meta-Research Innovation Center (METRIC) at Stanford University to improve the validity and reproducibility of scientific studies by organizing conferences and by monitoring scientific publications.

One reason for this state of affairs is that studies do not give enough information to permit accurate replication of them. Another, probably more important reason is the competitiveness of science. As the ranks of active researchers have swelled, scientists have lost their taste for self-policing and quality control. The competitive obligation to "publish or perish" has come to rule academic life. Ioannidis points out that that every year six freshly minted Ph.D.s vie for every academic post. It's come to the point where the replication of other researchers' results does little to advance a researcher's career. And without being refuted, dubious findings live on to mislead.

What's more, because too many researchers are chasing a dwindling pot of research money, Harold Varmus, Director of the National Cancer Institute, said: "Our whole system of operating is basically one that is probably not sustainable. That is, the idea that we're going to be able to fund more and more people, train a lot of people and expand to meet all of the opportunities that are there scientifically just does not accord with the current economic situation."[6] Varmus also wants to address what he calls the "flawed values system" that the competitive atmosphere of cancer research has spawned. The result is an "insidious and pervasive problem of people and labs competing for jobs, grants, etc." He noted that encouraging openness among researchers could help.

In addition, the research priorities have been focused on themes that have turned out to be flawed and unproductive. The most obvious is the emphasis placed on the genetic aspects of cancer.

Cancer Genomics

On April 14, 2003, scientists announced they had completed the multi-billion dollar Human Genome Project by compiling a list of the three trillion letters of the genetic code that make up what they considered to be a model of everyone's DNA. This generalized genome, which is 99.9% identical in each one of us, has become the tool for research in a variety of venues, especially cancer that does have genetic components.

The experience of Elaine Mardis and her colleagues at Washington University School of Medicine in St. Louis is worth noting. They were not content to sequence the genes of just one patient or even one cancer.[7] They got in on the ground floor of the Cancer Genome Atlas, a massive National Institutes of Health (NIH) effort to describe the molecular basis of twenty cancers.[8] They use technology to find genes and pathways across many tumors that may work as drug targets and to see how tumors develop resistance to treatment.

Mardis' team helped save the life of one of their colleagues after he relapsed with acute myelogenous leukemia (AML). By providing him with what Mardis called the Maserati approach—a series of genetic analyses that she hopes may one day become standard for clinical care—they identified an existing drug that stopped his relapse in its tracks.

In 2007 Mardis proposed a project, estimated to cost $1 million, to NIH as part of their grant renewal, but the study section reviewing it "hated it," Mardis recalls. Unfazed, they pitched their case to a local philanthropist, Alvin J. Siteman, after whom Washington University's cancer center is named. Their resulting article, published in *Nature* in 2008, was an eye-opener followed by ongoing clinical trials.[9] The team pinpointed 10 relevant gene mutations, two of which were already linked to AML, and eight that were new to oncologists. This started the idea of doing a personal genetic profile for each cancer patient. For eight AML patients, the Washington University group sequenced cancer cells when each person was first diagnosed and when the patient relapsed after chemotherapy. The relapse cancer came from the same pool of bone marrow cells that had led to cancer in the first place, but those cells had undergone additional mutations. "We were the first to confirm what was suspected for some time. By using chemotherapy, we may be setting up the patient to relapse because of acquired new mutations," said Mardis.[10]

This observation also was made by oncologist Charles Swanton who too often must tell his patients with advanced lung and breast cancer their options are running out.[11] Despite several different treatments, each somewhat successful at first, their tumors grew back yet again, faster than ever. "It's as though tumors have this ability to guess what you are about to do next and preempt it," he lamented. Tumors were long thought to evolve in a linear fashion as a single cell acquired growth-spurring mutations and dominated the final mass. But studies have shown that in many tumors cells branch off and form tumors with cells that evade treatments.

Genomic studies like Swanton's are stirring new interest in an old idea—tumors are a mosaic of different cells—by confirming with modern techniques that tumors are not always dominated by genetically identical cells, as once thought. Instead, tumors often contain many subsets of cells that are related but genetically distinct. As a tumor evolves, cells split off and develop new mutations or other errors, like a tree growing many branches. This means that two parts of the same tumor, as well as the metastases that form when that cancer spreads, look very different genetically.

The extent to which cells vary within a given tumor has shaken cancer biologists and clinicians. They're rethinking major projects to deal with cancer mutations because the current approach is based on a single cell type for each tumor. New studies suggest that the growing practice of analyzing the genetic and molecular characteristics of a single tumor biopsy to guide patient treatment is misleading. Cancer's heterogeneity could account for why new drugs that target specific gene mutations almost inevitably stop working. They merely give drug-resistant cells a chance to grow.

Both the promise and the problems with the genetic approach to cancer were illustrated in a Special Section on Breast Cancer in the March 28, 2014, issue of *Science* magazine.[12] Few scientific endeavors captured as much public interest as the race to identify *BRCA1*, a gene that protects women from breast and ovarian cancers. The search culminated in a 1994 *Science* article reporting the isolation of *BRCA1* with *BRCA2* being identified soon thereafter. Twenty years later, the *BRCA* genes continue to make headlines, sparking a 2013 U.S. Supreme Court decision banning patenting naturally occurring genes and intense debates on the ethics of genetic testing.

Widespread breast screening has led to early detection and a new dilemma: whether to aggressively treat non-cancerous lesions that may never become invasive or whether to "watch and wait." Since 1994, dozens more genes have been found that increase a woman's risk of hereditary breast cancer, but by how much is uncertain, confounding already complicated issues in genetic testing and counseling. There is no doubt that testing for *BRCA1* and *BRCA2* mutations in the past twenty years has saved lives. But these mutations account for only 5 to 10 percent of breast cancer cases, and breast cancer remains the most common and deadly cancer in women. Paula Kiberstis, Senior Editor of *Science*, asked: "Is it time to start a new race?"

Mary-Clair King, Professor of Genome Sciences and of Medicine at Washington University in St. Louis, commented: "A path that began nicely enough with two or three adjacent genes would soon turn back on itself, yielding more a meander through a swamp than a walk from one signpost to another."[13] Matthew Ellis, Professor of Medicine in the Oncology Division of Washington University, cautioned. "There's a moral hazard here. Just adding genetic information doesn't necessarily lead to better clinical management. A bad test can be as bad as a bad drug."[14]

Certain mutated genes cause cancer cells to proliferate uncontrollably, to spread to new tissues where they don't belong and to refuse to end their lives when they should. So research should revolve around finding first the mechanisms through which these mutated genes rise and second the drugs that can stop the resulting neoplastic process.

A 2014 review of 3,527 tumors representing 12 cancer types concluded that 10 percent of patients could find better therapies if they had information about their tumor's unique DNA and how it is expressed.[15]

Should You Have a Genetic Analysis?

Dr. Theodora Ross, director of the University of Texas Southwestern Medical Center Cancer Genetics Program, offered advice for people who want to know what their genes might tell them about their risks for cancer in a *The New York Times* article.[16] She said, first, it's important to know the difference between analyzing a tumor and analyzing a germ line. The germ line genome is found in every cell of the body and encodes traits such as eye color and the tendency to develop diseases like cystic fibrosis. It's the blueprint you inherited from your parents. The tumor genome is like an ugly addition on top of the original construction. It's acquired rather than inherited and contains a mess of new mutations, a subset of which causes the cells to proliferate out of control and transform into cancer. It's unclear how many people would benefit from analyzing all the genes in a tumor; it, like full germ line analysis, remains mainly a research tool.

The genetic tests that are clearly valuable at this point for predicting cancer risk are those for the specific mutations that are understood. But even then there can be other mutations in the same genes that are of unknown clinical significance. So the best results come from analyzing the subset of genes that could potentially explain patterns of disease observed in a family tree. If your family shows an increased incidence of certain cancers, it makes sense to look for known mutations that increase the risk of those cancers.

For example, Dr. Ross saw a 25-year-old patient with a strong family history of colon cancer. His father had colon cancer. When the son tested positive for a broken colon cancer gene, the rest of his family followed. Those who tested positive now know they need to have frequent colonoscopies. And most people with strong family histories of breast cancer should consider getting genetic counseling and, if recommended, testing for mutations in genes such as PALB2, BRCA1 and BRCA2.

For any patient who still wants to get his or her full genome sequenced, Dr. Ross said there is one good reason to do it: scientific curiosity. Something of interest could come of it as the technology improves over time. But it's worth doing only if a clinical trial is paying for it, or if you can easily afford it. Getting the data can cost under $2,000, but having the data interpreted can cost in the tens or hundreds of thousands of dollars. It's a fine purchase, but definitely a luxury. And bear in mind that the data that come back will raise more questions than they answer. There is a good chance that mutations of unknown clinical significance will be found that will increase anxiety without illuminating any known risks. Dr. Ross concluded that most people should focus less on the high-tech future of genetic testing and more on the low-tech history of their family trees.

A Lack of Focus on Metastasis

All of this must be viewed in the context of the likelihood that genetic research will not lead to treatments with enduring benefits because of the ability of cancer cells to mutate and evade genetically based interventions. That's because when most malignant solid tumors are diagnosed, there's a strong chance that some of those cells with different genetic characteristics have already broken off from the initial tumor and are on their way to another part of the body through metastasis.

Most of those cells will not take root in another tissue or organ. A metastasizing cell has an uphill battle to survive once it enters the violent churn of the bloodstream. But the process has begun—and with a billion cells dividing like there's no tomorrow, an ever-growing number of cancer cells will make the journey. Inevitably, many will succeed.

In the end, it's not localized tumors that kill people with cancer; it's metastasis. Aggressive cells spread to the liver, lungs, brain and other vital areas, wreaking havoc. So you'd think that cancer researchers would have been bearing down on this insidious phenomenon of metastasis over the years instead of just focusing on shrinking tumors. Clifton Leaf pointed out that, according to a *Fortune* magazine examination of National Cancer Institute (NCI) grants going back to 1972, less than 0.5 percent of study proposals focused primarily on metastasis. Of nearly 8,900 NCI grant proposals awarded in 2012, 92 percent didn't even mention the word metastasis.[17]

One accomplished researcher sent an elegant proposal to the NCI to study the epigenetics (changes in the gene's environment) of metastases vs. primary tumors. It's now in its third resubmission, he said to Leaf. "I mean, there is nothing known about that. But somehow I can't interest people in funding this!"

M.D. Anderson Cancer Center's Isaiah Fidler suggested to Leaf that metastasis is getting short shrift simply because "it's tough. Okay? And individuals are not rewarded for doing tough things. Grant reviewers are more comfortable with focused experiments that generate easily reproducible results." Fidler is right. Metastasis is a body-wide phenomenon that may involve dozens of processes. It's hard to do replicable experiments when there are that many variables. But that's the kind of research we need.

The drive to accumulate easily reproducible data also goes to the heart of the regulatory process for drug development. The Food and Drug Administration's mandate is to make sure that a drug is safe and that it works before allowing its sale to the public. Thus, regulators need to see hard data showing that a drug has had some effect when tested. This means that clinical trials have to be based on patients with obvious tumors that can be measured. It's hard to see cancer cells spreading throughout a body, although it actually can be done now by counting cancer cells and the breakdown products of DNA through newly evolved technologies.

Leaf concluded that pharma companies, quite naturally, don't concentrate on solving the problem of metastasis (the thing that kills people); they focus on devising drugs that shrink tumors (the things that don't kill but can be easily observed to shrink).

Research on Mice

Another problem in research is that a mouse gene may be very similar to a human gene, but the rest of the mouse is very different. The fact that so many cancer researchers seem to forget or ignore this observation when working with mouse models in the lab clearly irks Robert Weinberg. A professor of biology at MIT and winner of the National Medal of Science for his discovery of both the first human oncogene and the first tumor-suppressor gene, Weinberg told Leaf that one of the most frequently used experimental models of human cancer is to take human cancer cells that are grown in a petri dish, put them in a mouse that's immune system has been compromised, allow them to form a tumor and then expose the mouse to different kinds of drugs that might be useful in treating people. These are called "preclinical models".

Weinberg added that it's been well known for more than a decade that many of these preclinical human cancer models have very little predictive power in terms of how actual human tumors inside patients will respond. "Despite the genetic and organ-system similarities between a mouse and a human," he says, "the two species have key differences in physiology, tissue architecture, metabolic rate, immune system function, molecular signaling, you name it. So the tumors that arise in each, with the same flip of a genetic switch, are vastly different. A fundamental problem which remains to be solved in the whole cancer research effort, in terms of therapies, is that the preclinical models of human cancer, in large part, stink."

Bruce Chabner, a professor of medicine at Harvard and clinical director at the Massachusetts General Hospital Cancer Center, also told Leaf that he finds the mouse models lacking. He explained that for a variety of biological reasons the "instant tumors" that researchers cause in mice simply can't mimic human cancer's most critical and maddening trait—its quickly-changing DNA. That characteristic leads to staggering complexity in the most deadly tumors.

"If you find a compound that cures hypertension in a mouse, it's going to work in people. We don't know how toxic it will be, but it will probably work," said Chabner, who for many years ran the cancer treatment division at the NCI. "So researchers routinely try the same approach with cancer, 'knocking out' this gene or 'knocking in' that one in a mouse and causing a tumor to appear. Then they say, 'I've got a model for lung cancer!' Well, it ain't a model for lung cancer, because lung cancer in humans has a hundred mutations. It looks like the most complicated thing you've ever seen genetically."

Homer Pearce, who once ran cancer research and clinical investigation at Eli Lilly, agrees that mouse models are "woefully inadequate" for determining whether a drug will work in humans. "If you look at the millions and millions of mice that have been cured, and you compare that to the relative success, or lack thereof, that we've achieved in the treatment of metastatic disease clinically," he said to Leaf, "you realize that there just has to be something wrong with those models."

Vishva Dixit, a vice president for research in molecular oncology at Genentech in South San Francisco, is even more horrified that 99% of investigators in industry and in academia use xenografts (cross species models). "Why is the mouse model so heavily used? Simple. It's very convenient, easily manipulated," Dixit explained to Leaf. "You can assess tumor size just by looking at it."

Although drug companies clearly recognize the problem, they haven't fixed it. And they'd better, Weinberg added, "if for no other reason than hundreds of millions of dollars are being wasted every year by drug companies using these models."

Even more discouraging is the very real possibility that reliance on this flawed model has caused researchers to pass over drugs that would work in humans. After all, if so many promising drugs that clobbered mouse cancers failed in humans, the reverse also is likely too. More than a few of the hundreds of thousands of compounds discarded over the past 20 years might have been effective agents in human beings.

Roy Herbst, who divides his time between laboratory bench and bedside at M.D. Anderson and who has run trials on Iressa and other targeted therapies for lung cancer, is sure that happens often. "It's something that bothers me a lot," he said to Leaf. "We probably lose a lot of things that either don't have activity on their own, or we haven't tried in the right setting, or you don't identify the right target."

"If everyone understands there's a problem, why isn't anything being done? Two understandable reasons," said Weinberg. "First, there's no other model to replace that poor mouse. Second, the FDA has created inertia because it continues to recognize these models as the gold standard for predicting the utility of drugs."

Leaf asks one of the many chicken-and-egg questions bedeviling the cancer culture. Which came first: the FDA's imperfect standards for judging drugs or the pharmaceutical companies' imperfect models for testing them? The riddle is applicable not just to early drug development in which flawed animal models fool scientists into thinking their new compounds will wallop tumors in humans. It comes up with far more important ramifications in the last stage of human testing when the FDA is looking for signs that a new drug is actually helping the patients who are taking it.

It's exciting to see a tumor shrink in a mouse or human and know that a drug is doing that. A shrinking tumor is intuitively a good thing. So it is no surprise that it's one of the key goals in most clinical trials. That's in no small part because it's a measurable goal: we can see it happening. When you read the word "response" in a newspaper story about some exciting new cancer drug, tumor shrinkage is what it's talking about.

But Leaf noted that tumor regression by itself actually is a lousy predictor for the progression of disease. Oncologists often can shrink a tumor with chemotherapy and radiotherapy. That sometimes makes the cancer easier to remove surgically. If not, it still may buy time. However, if the doctors don't get every cancer cell, the sad truth is that the tumor regression is not likely to improve the person's chances of survival.

Still research on animals remains a mainstay of medical research to the extent that it can be translated into clinical applications in human beings.

Basic Science vs Translational Research

On the positive side, the past decade has brought together substantial advances in human genome analysis and an understanding of tumor biology, but often it's difficult to apply this information to patients. For example, National Cancer Institute (NCI) scientists have directly observed events that lead to the formation of a chromosome abnormality that often is found in cancer cells.[18] The abnormality, called a translocation, occurs when part of a chromosome breaks off and becomes attached to another chromosome. It's long been known that translocations play a role in cancer development. However, despite many years of research, exactly how translocations form in a cell remains a mystery. This may change as NCI scientists now are able to visualize translocations in real time and to observe changes in thousands of cells over long time periods and apply this knowledge to solve clinical problems.

Georgetown University oncologist John L. Marshall noted that the lion's share of our research dollar is going to basic science.[19] "These are the animal and Petri dish models. Time and again, we see that the basic science models do not reflect what happens in the clinic. We must get away from spending all of this money on basic science research and shift it to research on patients. The patient is the only model in which we will learn how to cure cancer. In every case of molecular targeted therapies, it's the patient who has taught us the molecular biology—not the molecular biologist. The latter has been an incredibly inefficient and misdirected use of our research dollars. We should shift that funding over to innovative clinical translational research, where we embrace the complexity of our patients and their tumors, figure out how to measure a moving target, and not continue the static long-term model that has been stable for twenty-five years in someone's lab. We have to figure that out in the patient and not in the lab."

Unstable and Inadequate Research Funding

Money fuels research and biomedical scientists in the United States have been buffeted by the funding swings of the National Institutes of Health (NIH), their field's primary benefactor. They're anxious about the future, as Congress tries to rein in debt by slowing government spending.[20] As a result, morale is as low and uncertainty as high as she's ever seen it according to molecular biologist Shirley Tilghman, president emerita of Princeton University. "The image that comes into my head is a seesaw," she said. "The highs are higher and the lows are lower. The NIH's budget's wild swings make for an inefficient research enterprise."

"The fundamental problems are structural in nature," concluded Michael Teitelbaum of the Alfred P. Sloan Foundation in New York City back in 2008. "Biomedical research funding is both erratic and subject to positive-feedback loops that together drive the system ineluctably toward damaging instability."

What's more, few new bold projects are being funded. Clifton Leaf noted that in 2010, the National Cancer Institute used the bulk of its $1.8 billion in research grants on existing projects.[21] In 2011, the top 43 research centers got more funding than did the bottom 2,574 institutions receiving any kind of NIH support. To some, this is the price of science that is both sound and safe. To others, it is a culture of scientific inefficiency, an "IBM mindset" in a field that desperately yearns for "Apple."

Even more ominous is the fact that the National Science Foundation awarded 1,000 fewer grants in 2013 than in the previous year. Bruce Alberts, Editor-in-Chief of the prestigious scientific journal *Science* asks: Are we headed for a future where the world's most talented young scientists no longer want to pursue careers in the United States?[22]

Individual Ingenuity—Productive or Not?

Here is an example of a discovery that did not involve an institution or funding. After a family friend died of pancreatic cancer, high school sophomore Jack Andraka invented a simple diagnostic strip that could detect that kind of cancer in its early stages in the spring of 2011.[23]

After reading up on the disease, Andraka discovered that around 85 percent of pancreatic cancers are diagnosed too late, when patients have less than a 2 percent chance of survival. The reason, he learned, was that the best tools for early detection are both expensive and woefully inaccurate.

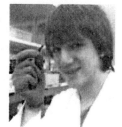

Jack Andraka

A typical teenager might have left it there, but Andraka dove deeply into the scientific literature. He learned about a popular biomarker called mesothelin—a protein in the blood that's overexpressed in patients with several types of cancer, including pancreatic cancer, even in the earliest stages. Andraka also was thinking about carbon nanotubes—tiny cylinders, around 1/50,000 the diameter of a human hair, with amazing mechanical and electrical properties, which he described as "the superheroes of materials science."

Then, while learning about antibodies in biology class, Andraka was struck with an idea. He thought maybe if he laced mesothelin-specific antibodies into a network of carbon nanotobes he could change the network's electrical properties based on the amount of the antibody present—a signal detectable with a simple ohmmeter.

Andraka wrote up a detailed research proposal and e-mailed it to scientists at Johns Hopkins University (JHU) and the National Institutes of Health. He received a raft of rejections—and one maybe, from Anirban Maitra, a pathologist at JHU. "It was remarkable because he sent a very specific, 30-page protocol including reagents and pitfalls and everything," said Maitra, who, after meeting (and grilling) Andraka, invited the teenager to work in his lab.

By January 2012, Andraka's dedication was beginning to pay off. In a series of pilot studies, he demonstrated that his dip-coated filter paper test strips—hooked up via electrodes to a $50 ohmmeter from Home Depot—were capable of measuring mesothelin levels in the blood of mice with pancreatic tumors and in a limited number of human serum samples.

Andraka's work won him the grand prize at the 2012 Intel International Science and Engineering Fair in Pittsburgh, which came with $75,000 in scholarships. Maitra said he was sure his young protégé would achieve great things. "He's a remarkable kid," Maitra said. "Whatever he goes into, he will excel, but hopefully we can keep him in biomedical science."

While the media version is glowing, an alternative version of the Andraka story is more chastening.[24] Unfortunately, what was portrayed in the media as an inspired break through has not been published in any paper clearly outlining Andraka's methods or findings. His claims have yet to be replicated. He may be a young man overwhelmed by big science, big business and big fame and who is not following scientific protocols regarding publication and peer review.

Whatever the final version of the Andraka story ends up being, it's clear that the story is far from settled. In the final analysis, it could all be for naught and once again illustrate the vagaries of cancer research, or it could be successful and encourage others to follow their dreams. In either event, the mass media and enthusiasts typically get ahead of the facts.

Conclusion

With the plummeting cost of genomic analysis, one can envision a day in the near future when a complete cancer genetic profile and other molecular evaluations becomes a standard component of an initial diagnostic evaluation. Patients will be armed with molecular information about their own tumors, and thus able to make more informed decisions about treatment. Still, translating this information into practical clinical applications remains slow.

It's likely that genetic research will not lead to treatments with enduring benefits because of the ability of cancer cells to mutate and evade genetically based interventions. By the time a tumor is discovered, there is a strong chance that some of those mutated cells are on their way to another part of the body through metastasis.

A major contribution of genetic research is a shift in the focus of routine cancer treatment from the organ of origin to the genetic profile of the cancer. This fundamental goal—to be able to read the complex code embedded in our bodies in order to identify the best therapies for each individual over the entire course of treatment—portends a medical breakthrough. It also may make it possible to identify persons at risk for developing cancer.

With an understanding of its limitations, research on animal models of physiological systems and cancer treatments is a major tool in preclinical research. The key is translating and applying research to the actual treatment of human beings.

Chapter Seven

Testing Treatments

The pros and cons of current clinical trials for testing the effectiveness of cancer treatments are described.

The Pharmaceutical Research and Manufacturers of America (PhRMA) represents the country's leading pharmaceutical industry research and biotechnology companies. It's devoted to inventing medicines that allow patients to live longer, healthier and more productive lives. It holds that PhRMA companies are leading the way in the search for new cures for cancer.

PhRMA points out that America's biopharmaceutical research sector is the global leader in medical innovation with more than three hundred new medicines approved by the Food and Drug Administration in the last decade. In 2012 America's biopharma research companies were testing 981 medicines and vaccines to fight the many types of cancer.[1] These medicines were either in clinical trials or awaiting review by the Food and Drug Administration.

Novartis is a major player in pharmaceutical research. A Novartis executive was interviewed by *Fortune* magazine in 2013.[2] He said that oncology will be going through an era of medical breakthroughs in pharmaceutical development in the next 5 to 10 years. He added that the deep sequencing of the human genome has created a wealth of data that will allow new areas of discovery that have never been possible before. The executive concluded by stating that Novartis is unlike most pharmaceutical companies because ten years ago it started a pathways approach, which is devoted to understanding the molecular pathway of a particular form of cancer.

There will be a rise in the number of trials that incorporate molecular tumor testing prior to treatment with treatment selection based on the molecular features of each individual's cancer. Such personalized trials have the potential to yield better outcomes by increasing the probability of response and to employ less toxic therapies by increasingly targeting cancer-specific functions, rather than all cells that are growing rapidly.

This shift in the way clinical trials are conducted is the result of dissatisfaction with the present system. In his 2003 *Fortune* magazine article, Clifton Leaf noted that a blue-ribbon panel of cancer-center directors concluded then that clinical trials are "long, arduous," and burdened with regulations.[3] Without major change and better resources, the panel concluded, the "system is likely to remain inefficient, unresponsive and unduly expensive." All that patients know is that the process has little to offer them as illustrated by the fact that 97% of adults with cancer don't participate in clinical trials.

Costs of Clinical Trials

Because of the duration and cost of clinical trials, drug companies that sponsor the vast majority of them have an overwhelming incentive to test drugs that are likely to win Food and Drug Administration approval. After all, they are public companies with shareholders expecting a return on their investments. So they focus not on breakthrough treatments but on incremental improvements to existing classes of drugs. The process does not encourage innovation or entrepreneurial approaches to drug discovery. It does not encourage brave new thinking. Not when testing a drug typically takes at least five to ten years.

In 1975, the pharmaceutical industry spent the equivalent of $100 million in today's dollars for research and development of the average drug approved by the Food and Drug Administration, according to the Tufts Center for the Study of Drug Development. By 1987 that figure had tripled to $300 million. By 2005, the 1987 figure had more than quadrupled to $1.3 billion.[4] According to *Forbes* magazine, partly because so many drugs fail large pharmaceutical companies that are working on dozens of drug projects at once may spend a staggering $5 billion for each new medicine that is approved.[5]

There are two kinds of costs associated with clinical trials: patient care costs and research costs.

1) Patient care costs fall into two categories:
   + Usual care costs, such as doctor visits, hospital stays, clinical laboratory tests and x-rays, which occur whether you are participating in a trial or receiving standard treatment. These costs usually are covered by a third-party health plan, such as Medicare or private insurance.
   + Extra care costs associated with clinical trial participation, such as the additional tests that may or may not be fully covered by the clinical trial sponsor and/or research institution. The clinical trial sponsor and the participant's health plan need to resolve coverage of these costs for particular trials.
2) Research costs are those associated with conducting the trial, such as data collection and management, research physician and nurse time, analysis of results and tests purely performed for research purposes. Such costs are usually covered by the sponsoring organization, such as the National Cancer Institute or a pharmaceutical company. These costs are not the patient's responsibility.

What's more, the system essentially forces companies to test the most promising new compounds on the sickest patients—where it is easy to see some activity (like shrinking tumors) but almost impossible to cure people. At that point the disease has typically spread too far, and the tumors have become too ridden with genetic mutations. So drugs that might have worked well in earlier-stage patients often never get a chance to be tested.

Another problem is that clinical trials are focused on the wrong goal—on doing "proper" science rather than saving lives. It's not that they provide bad care—patients in trials are treated especially well. But a trial's purpose is to test a hypothesis: Is treatment X better than treatment Y? And sometimes the information generated by this tortuously long process doesn't matter much. If you've spent ten years to discover that a new drug shrinks a tumor by an average of 10% more than the existing standard of care, how many people have you really helped?

Examples of Clinical Trials

Clifton Leaf obtained information about two drugs approved for cancer of the colon and rectum: Avastin and Erbitux.[6] In each case it took many months just to enroll the necessary number of patients in clinical trials. Participating doctors then had to administer the drugs according to often arduous preset protocols, collecting reams of data along the way. After years of testing when Avastin was added to the standard chemotherapy regimen, the combination managed to extend the lives of some 400 patients with terminal colorectal cancer by a median 4.7 months. (A previous trial of the drug on breast cancer patients failed to extend lives at all.) This small gain was seen as substantial, considering that those in advanced stages of the disease typically live less than 16 months. Those who responded to the chemotherapy lived only 29% longer!

Although Erbitux did indeed shrink tumors, it has not been shown to prolong patients' lives at all. Some certainly fared well on the drug, but survival on average for the groups studied didn't change. Still, Erbitux was approved for use primarily in "third line" therapy, after every other accepted treatment has failed. A weekly dose costs $2,400.

Remember, it took several years and the participation of thousands of patients in three stages of testing, tons of data and huge expense to find out what the clinicians and researchers already knew in the earliest stage of human testing: Neither drug would benefit more than a handful of the some 57,000 people who will die of colorectal cancer each year.

Leaf found that one targeted drug that clearly isn't a goose egg is

Novartis's Gleevec, which has been shown to save lives as well as stifle tumors. The drug has a dramatic effect on an uncommon kind of leukemia called Chronic Myelogenous Leukemia (CML) and an even more rare stomach cancer named GIST. Early reports said it also seems to work to varying degrees in up to three other cancers. Gleevec's success has been held out as the "proof of principle" that the strategy we've followed in the War on Cancer all these years has been right.

But even Gleevec is not what it seems. First, CML is not a complicated cancer. In it, a single gene mutation causes a critical signaling mechanism to go awry. Gleevec ingeniously interrupts that deadly signal. Most common cancers have as many as five to ten different things going wrong. Second, even "simple" cancers get smarter. The cancer cells long exposed to the drug (which must be taken for life) mutate their way around the molecular signal that Gleevec blocks, building drug resistance.

No wonder cancer is so much more vexing than heart disease. Bob Cohen, senior director for commercial diagnostics at Genentech, said to Leaf, "Use a drug that does not destroy the tumor completely and the heterogeneity will evolve from the (surviving) cells and say, 'I don't give a damn! You can't screw me up with this stuff.' Suddenly you're squaring and cubing the complexity. That's where we are." And that's why the only chance is to attack the disease earlier—and on multiple fronts.

Obstacles in Clinical Trials

Leaf also spoke with M.D. Anderson's Len Zwelling, who oversees regulatory compliance for the center's 800-plus clinical trials, and his wife, Genie Kleinerman, who is chief of pediatrics there. They called attention to the legal barriers that seem to be growing out of control. It took no more than ten minutes for Kleinerman to tell three stories about trying to bring together different drug companies in clinical trials for kids with cancer. In the first attempt, the clinical trial took so long that the biotech startup went out of business. In the second, the lawyers haggled over liability concerns until both companies pulled out. The third, however, was the worst. There were two drugs that together seemed to jolt the immune system into doing a better job of targeting malignant cells of osteosarcoma, a bone cancer that occurs in children. "Working with the lawyers, it was just impossible," she said, "because each side wanted to own the rights to the combination!"

The reliance on prospective, randomized, controlled trials as the only way to justify clinical implementation is not practical and guarantees that new information will have a multi-year lag while studies are constructed, conducted and interpreted. There also is a disconnection between the funding bodies and the prioritization of a particular type of study in terms of financial commitment, clinical trial infrastructure and ability to rapidly enact new strategies.

In his book *The Cure in the Code*, Peter Huber gives a compelling account of how 21st-century medicine is being hampered by a regulatory regime built for the science of the 20th century.[7] The FDA still operates according to the requirements of the age of mass drugs and has evolved into a bureaucracy more concerned with avoiding risk than speeding the benefits of innovation to patients. Drug approvals still depend on large-scale trials that focus on statistical correlations to determine clinical efficacy. Too often, the FDA refuses to approve a new drug because it doesn't work for everyone, when the goal should be to find those patients for whom it *does* work.

Huber argues that the current clinical-trial model should be replaced by adaptive trials in which both patients and physicians would continually learn and modify treatments along the way. Information about the molecular processes being targeted and the outcomes of each patient's therapeutic regimen would be reported to a broadly accessible digital knowledge network, which other doctors and patients could use to guide their choice of therapies.

Because so few adult cancer patients participate in clinical trials now, far more patients are needed to carry out meaningful clinical trials in the future. This will be most important for treatments that target relatively rare forms of cancer; a large number of potential subjects will have to be screened to find a sufficient number who have the same target for the drug being tested.

The Clinical Pharmacogenetics Implementation Consortium

There have been several efforts to develop ways to build consensus and collaboration among institutions around applying genetic information to drug therapy. One such effort is the Clinical Pharmacogenetics Implementation Consortium (CPIC).[8]

CPIC believes that we are on the cusp of significant change in the structure of cancer clinical trials as the emphasis shifts from large-scale studies of a drug on patients with similar diagnoses to smaller studies testing more targeted therapies in patients with similar cancer cell characteristics.[9] The previous generation of trials established the cancer treatment standards used today. CPIC envisions future cancer clinical trials that will be very different from those of the past with a more personalized, precise approach.

New Drug Development Paradigms

The New Drug Development Paradigms (NEWDIGS) is a collaborative effort that began at the Massachusetts Institute of Technology and includes representatives from drug regulators, drug companies, payers, patient organizations and academic institutions.[10] NEWDIGS's objective is to reliably and sustainably deliver new, better and affordable drugs to the right patients faster, and to counter "Pharmageddon," described by Hans-Georg Eichler, senior medical officer at the European Medicines Agency, as the "innovation engine, particularly in the biopharmaceutical industry, that isn't humming along as it should be. Everybody is a bit disgruntled and dissatisfied, whether you're a patient, in pharma, a provider, a payer or a regulator."

NEWDIGS was designed to provide a collaborative environment for innovation and learning that is creative and non-bureaucratic, taps the entrepreneurship and collective intelligence of its participants and has a collaborative impact similar to what the SEMATECH collaboration had on the semiconductor industry in the 1980s. NEWDIGS calls itself not just a "think tank" but also a "do tank".

NEWDIGS takes a systems approach to catalyzing change by exploring the co-evolution of processes, technologies, policies and people. NEWDIGS has developed the concept of adaptive licensing to counter some of the problems currently experienced with the regulation of new drugs.[11] According to Eichler, these problems stem in part from gradually learning about the effects of new drugs in a limited number of animals and people that occurs pre-clinically and during clinical testing. But "the next morning after that 'magic moment' when the new drug is approved, it's out the door and anyone can have it and we have no idea what happens to these patients. Is that wise?" Eichler asks.

Another problem is that some patient groups are frustrated that new drugs are not offered sooner to them, while some consumer advocates maintain that more needs to be known about drugs before they enter the market. Food and Drug Administration Commissioner Margaret Hamburg noted that the FDA has just "two speeds of approvals—too fast and too slow."[12]

To counter both problems, NEWDIGS has proposed doing away with the "magic moment" by creating a number of milestones where the data on the drug is looked at repeatedly over time; where the way a drug becomes available is aligned with growing knowledge and where uncertainty is progressively reduced. "We can broaden the access of the drug this way," Eichler explained. He noted that currently after a drug is licensed whether or not it works in practice is not followed. In contrast, with adaptive licensing after initial licensing of a drug the patient experience is captured, contributing information about the actual safety and effectiveness of the drug.

Unlike clinical trials that have strict conditions for patient participation, adaptive licensing studies have the advantage of better detecting drug effects in the "real world" when they are combined with other medications or affected by concomitant conditions. Eichler stressed, "We have to have the full spectrum of evidence-generation methodologies at our disposal, and you especially will need rapid learning systems in oncology where you probably have more variables than you have patients. The more information you can gather from the real world, the faster the learning experience will be."

Yale University Open Data Access Project

Traditionally, patient data that can be used to assess medical treatments has not been made available to researchers outside of an industry. As a result, independent researchers who are interested in evaluating a product have relied on data summaries and published manuscripts, which often provide an incomplete picture because much of the data is not published. The Yale University Open Data Access Project's (YODA) goal is to promote clinical trial data access more widely in order to increase transparency, to protect against industry influence and to accelerate the generation of new knowledge.[13]

The YODA Project model provides a means for the rigorous and objective evaluation of clinical trial data to ensure that patients and physicians possess all the necessary information about a drug or device when making treatment decisions. This process includes both coordinating independent examinations of all relevant product data by two separate qualified research groups and making all patient-level clinical research data available for analysis by other external investigators. The model is designed to provide industry with confidence that the analyses will be scientifically rigorous, objective and fair.

Compassionate Access to Unapproved Drugs

Because the pace of clinical trials can be so slow, patients have successfully argued for "compassionate access" to unapproved drugs. But not all companies willingly allow compassionate access to drugs in their pipelines. Only 6 percent of early-stage cancer drugs ever come to market because many are found to have severe side effects or just don't work.[14] Given these odds, companies hesitate to do anything to jeopardize a product too soon. If they give drugs away, a disastrous side effect or other poor outcomes could spur bad publicity and extra scrutiny from regulators.

Even more importantly, if doctors simply let people take untested medicines without going through clinical trials, drug companies would have difficulty getting anyone to enroll in them, getting the data on safety and efficacy for FDA approval and passing the gateway to big sales. "Even if patients with cancer are willing buyers, drug manufacturers are not willing sellers." said George Annas, a Boston University expert on medical law.[15]

If we simply let people have access to untested medicines without trials, we will never learn which ones are effective and how best to use them. But to a physician face-to-face with desperate patients, the case for the greater good seems less compelling. After all, the promising drug may be the patient's last and only chance. Now and then desperation leads to obtaining a drug through the compassionate use policy and is successful.

Still, access to unproven medicines cannot be an absolute right. It must depend on review by an experienced doctor who can weigh complex medical data to make educated guesses about what to do. Otherwise, patients can be vulnerable to charlatans.

Provocative Issues

Europe has taken the lead in adopting measures to ensure openness of data collected through drug trials. In 2014 the European Parliament voted to require that clinical trial results be published within a year of completion, whether or not the data are positive.[16] Since 2007 the U. S. Food and Drug Administration has required drug makers to post some trial results in the government registry within a year of a drug's approval, but a 2012 study showed that fewer than one in four approved drugs had results that were filed in time.

In March 2014, the American Society of Clinical Oncology released *Raising the Bar for Clinical Trials by Defining Clinically Meaningful Outcomes*, which calls on the community of patients, patient advocates and clinical investigators to collectively raise the bar in expectations of the benefits of new therapies and to design clinical trials to demonstrate greater benefits.[17]

It is striking to note that although there are many claims of cancer cures, they seldom are reported in reputable professional journals that specialize in case reports, such as Wiley's *Clinical Case Reports*. More specifically, the "n of one" is a scientifically acceptable experimental model. This simply involves collecting data on the effects of treatment on an individual person and publishing it in a credible scientific format. In fact the "n of one" approach is valid when a dramatic result is demonstrated in changes from before to after the course of treatment. This type of study has enabled practitioners to achieve experimental progress without the overwhelming work of designing a group comparison study. It can effectively suggest causality if a problem vanished during the treatment.

Another option is to adapt the current clinical trial model for cancer to specific circumstances. As it now stands, there are four potential phases in cancer clinical trials:

1) Initial trial of a drug in humans for dosing, safety and early efficacy information (20-80 patients)
2) Subsequent trial of a drug's safety and efficacy in a particular disease setting (100-300 patients)
3) Larger trial comparing a drug with best available therapy to confirm efficacy and safety; often used for drug approval (1,000-3,000 patients)
4) Trial conducted after Food and Drug Administration approval to gain additional information about the drug's risks and benefits (thousands of patients)

Why couldn't phase 1) be continued as the clinical trial with appropriate safety adjustments if a drug appears to be efficacious until its actual benefit can be ascertained?

Conclusion

Because of the duration and cost of clinical trials, drug companies have an overwhelming incentive to test compounds that are likely to win Food and Drug Administration approval. So they have focused on incremental improvements to existing classes of drugs rather than on breakthrough treatments.

The reliance on prospective, randomized, controlled trials as the only way to justify clinical implementation has proved to be impractical and guarantees that new information usually will have a five- to ten-year lag while trials are constructed, conducted and interpreted.

The New Drug Development Paradigms is a collaborative effort that includes representatives from drug regulators, drug companies, payers, patient organizations and academic institutions. This endeavor's objective is to deliver new, better and affordable drugs to the right patients faster by taking a systems approach through adaptive licensing to counter some of the problems currently experienced with the regulation of clinical trials.

Oncology will be going through an era of breakthroughs in pharmaceutical development. There will be a rise in the number of trials that incorporate molecular tumor testing prior to treatment with treatment selection based on the molecular features of each individual's cancer. Such personalized trials have the potential to yield better outcomes by increasing the probability of a positive response and to employ less toxic therapies by increasingly targeting cancer-producing functions rather than all rapidly growing cells.

Chapter Eight

Changing the Way We Think About Cancer

New approaches to cancer are reactivating long known, and trying out new, ideas and methods.

The sun rises and the sun sets. It seems like the sun rotates around the Earth. Cancer cells rise and are killed by surgery, radiation and chemotherapy. It seems like cancer is a disease. But the sun does not rotate around the Earth, and cancer is not a disease. The many kinds of cancer cells are the products of the disease *neoplasia* that can emerge in our bodies' organs and tissues.

Strange as it may seem, much of the failure of the War on Cancer—and more importantly, much of the potential for finally winning it—has to do with the definition of cancer.

In a 2013 *Time* magazine article, Bill Saporito described cancer as "not just one disease; it's hundreds, potentially thousands. And not all cancers are caused by just one agent—a virus or bacterium that can be flushed and crushed. Cancer is an intricate and potentially lethal collaboration of genes gone awry, of growth inhibitors gone missing, of hormones and epigenomes changing and rogue cells breaking free. It works as one great armed force, attacking by the equivalent of air and land and sea and stealth, and we think we're going to take it out with what? A lab-coated sniper?"[1] This image of cancer as a myriad of diseases makes cancer seem unconquerable.

In contrast, if we think of cancer as a complicated array of conditions arising from the dysfunctional bodily process of neoplasia, it makes it easier to organize research and treatment around preventing and stopping that process. The journal *Neoplasia* does this by encompassing the traditional disciplines of cancer research as well as emerging fields and interdisciplinary investigations. Cancer remains a daunting challenge, but at least we have conceptual clarity now to guide us rather than overwhelming confusion.

To simplify the matter, killing cancer cells is like using insulin to lower the blood sugar levels in diabetes. Both cancer cells and high blood sugar are products of underlying diseases: cancer cells of neoplasia and high blood sugar of deficient insulin production by the Isles of Langerhans cells of the pancreas in type 1 diabetes. Incidentally, scientists at the University of North Carolina School of Medicine and the City of Hope National Medical Center are opening the door to treating the cause of diabetes by showing that injections of certain antibodies reinvigorated the Isle of Langerhans cells and reversed the onset of Type I diabetes in mice genetically bred to develop the disease.[2] Moreover, just two injections in the North Carolina study maintained disease remission indefinitely without harming the immune system.

Although proposed in 1957 and subsequent decades, only recently has the focus of cancer research been shifting to why there is a lapse in our bodies' natural defenses in our immune systems that ordinarily detect and destroy abnormal cells. That lapse permits cancer cells to grow and spread.

The major focus of cancer treatment has been on "search for and destroy cancer cells." It has been on destroying cancer cells...not on preventing or stopping their formation. Tumors are identified and surgery, radiation and/or chemotherapy are used to eliminate cancer cells. In the process, especially with radiation and chemotherapy, normal growing cells are destroyed as well, and the body's natural defense system—the immune system—is compromised. This model relies upon the fallacy that medical interventions can cure a disease without the help of our bodies' natural defenses. Most importantly, it focuses on the products of a disease—cancer cells—rather than on the disease itself...neoplasia.

A more realistic and productive model is based on the fact that our normal body cells are continuously changing and, if in that process do not die normally, can mutate through a process called neoplasia and become cancer cells.

Preventing Neoplasia

Some 2,400 years ago the Greek physician Hippocrates described cancer as spreading out and grabbing on to another part of the body like "the arms of a crab," as he elegantly put it. Similarly, a popular view is that cancer begins when the cells of an expanding tumor push through the thin membrane that separates them from other tissues. It's a fancy way of saying that in order to become cancer, a cell has to go beyond its normal boundaries.

"Absolute nonsense!" said Michael Sporn, a professor of pharmacology and medicine at Dartmouth Medical School.[3] He went on: "We've been stuck with this definition of what cancer is from 1890. It's what I was taught in medical school: 'It's not cancer until there's invasion.' That's like saying the barn isn't on fire until there are bright red flames coming out of the roof."

In fact, cancer begins much earlier than that. And therein lies the best strategy to contain it. Sporn advocates preventing cells from entering the deadly stage of becoming cancer cells in the first place. He has been struggling for many years to get fellow researchers to start thinking about cancer not as a thing but as a process, called carcinogenesis—neoplasia, a multistage process that goes through various cell transformations that can progress slowly or rapidly.

So intervention must occur earlier in the process of neoplasia. To do this, the medical community has to break away from the notion that people in an early stage of neoplasia are "healthy" and therefore shouldn't be treated. People are not healthy if they're on a path toward cancer.

If this seems radical and far-fetched, consider this. We've prevented millions of heart attacks and strokes by using the very same strategy. Sporn likes to point out that heart disease doesn't start with the heart attack; it starts way earlier with dietary factors and insulin that cause arterial plaque (hardening of the arteries). So we treat those. In the same way, a stroke doesn't start with a blood clot in the brain. It often starts with hypertension. So we treat that with both lifestyle changes and drugs. "Cardiovascular disease, of course, is nowhere near as complex as cancer is," he admits, "but the principle is the same." Sporn adds: "All these people who are obsessed with cures for cancer are being selfish by ignoring what could be done in terms of prevention."

Actually, this principle is being applied to a limited extent right now. A perfect example is the Pap smear, which detects precancerous changes in the cells of the cervix. That simple procedure, followed by the surgical removal of any lesions, has dropped the incidence and death rates from cervical cancer by 78% and 79%, respectively, since the practice began in the 1950s.[4] Over 170 million tests have been given worldwide. In countries where Pap smears aren't done, cervical cancer is a leading killer of women.

The same goes for colon cancer. Not every polyp (a growth in the colon's lining) goes on to become malignant and invasive. But colon cancers have to go through this abnormal step on their way to becoming deadly. The list of other pre-cancerous conditions goes on from Barrett's esophagus (a precursor to cancer there) to hyperkeratosis (precursor of skin cancer). Doctors already are doing this kind of prevention with some other cancers, but they need to do it much more.

Biomarkers of Neoplasia

Some complain that the telltale biomarkers of neoplasia, while getting more predictive, still are far from definitive, and that we should wait until we know more. Researchers in heart disease, meanwhile, have taken the opposite tack and been far more successful. Neither obesity nor hypertension guarantee future cardiovascular disease, but they're treated anyway.

A few cancer researchers have made great strides in finding early warning signs by looking for protein and DNA breakdown products—"neoplastic signatures"—in blood, urine or even skin swabs that can identify precancerous conditions and very early cancers that are likely to progress. For instance, Lance Liotta, former chief of pathology at the National Cancer Institute, has demonstrated that ovarian cancer can be detected by a high-tech blood test—one that identifies a unique "cluster pattern" of some 70 different proteins in a woman's blood.[5] "We've discovered a previously unknown ocean of markers," he said. "And it's potentially a mammoth lifesaver. With current drugs, early-stage ovarian cancer is more than 90% curable; late stage is 75% deadly. Early results on a protein test for pancreatic cancer are promising as well," said Liotta.

One test is available now that could be useful with most cancers. Blood DNA levels have been found to be significantly elevated in patients with esophageal cancer and to return to normal levels following complete surgical removal of the cancer. Persistently elevated blood DNA levels after surgery or levels that rise on follow-up indicate residual or recurrent cancer.[6] Since DNA damage is a characteristic of neoplasia, this test may have broad applications.

Yes, the strategy has costs. Some say wholesale testing of biomarkers and early lesions—many of which won't go on to become invasive cancers—would result in a huge burden for the healthcare system and lead to a wave of potentially dangerous surgeries to remove things that might never become lethal anyway. But the costs of not acting are much greater.

Models for Treatment Directed at Cancer Cells Themselves

Focusing on neoplasia alone is not sufficient for destroying cancer cells that already have gone through that process. For a patient to become "cancer free" anti-cancer agents must 1) eradicate the primary tumor, 2) eradicate any tumors at other body locations that have arisen via metastasis and 3) eradicate any circulating tumor cells that remain in the blood. An example of an agent that may do all three is 3-bromopyruvate (3BP) discovered in Dr. Peter Pedersen's laboratory at Johns Hopkins

University by Dr. Young Ko near the turn of the century.[7] Like a "Trojan horse" 3-BP enters the cells of animal cancer tumors, targets HK-2 and quickly dissipates their energy production factories (glycolysis and mitochondria) resulting in tumor destruction without harm to the animals. In addition, 3BP at a dosage that kills cancer cells has little or no effect on normal cells. Therefore, 3BP can be considered a member of a new class of anti-cancer agents that attack the metabolism of cancer cells forming through neoplasia.

Researchers at the Mayo Clinic in Florida have identified a number of agents—some already used in the clinic for different disorders—that may force shape-shifting in tumor cells to immobilize them and thus prevent metastasis.[8] The researchers found that a protein called Syx is key to determining how tumor cells migrate. When researchers removed Syx from the cancer cells, they lost their polarity—their leading and trailing edges—and morphed into a "fried egg" shape.

Investigate All Significant Leads

There is good reason to question claims of successful cancer treatment that fall outside of the established professional fields. Quackery thrives when people are desperate to find effective treatment for all diseases. At the same time there are many reasonable leads that might prove productive, such as nutritional therapies, which are employed in Europe and in the United States, and scorpion venom therapy, which is used in Latin America.

Strikingly, nutritional therapy for cancer described in Chapter Ten has not been subjected to clinical studies in the way that chemotherapies have. This is most unfortunate since patients have been deprived of nutritional adjustments that could be helpful to them or of solid advice regarding their lack of effectiveness.

An example of a specific agent that may be a harbinger of things to come in destroying cancer cells that have formed tumors is blue scorpion venom. This venom is widely used in Cuba and other South American countries to treat cancer. Cuba's state pharmaceutical company, Labiofam, produces a homeopathic version of scorpion venom called Vidatox, which may not be as effective as normal doses of the venom that have been used. A handful of countries have registered it for sale, but it has not been evaluated in peer-reviewed journals.[9] According to authoritative reviews by U. S. physicians, the Cuban health system merits attention as an example of a nationally integrated approach resulting in improved health status.[10] We should not need an elaborate clinical trial to give an indication of whether or not this venom works in the United States. One reputable oncologist could use it with ten patients as a preliminary trial.

Scorpion venom actually has been used in the United States for brain tumors in the form of a tumor paint that is a molecule derived from the venom consisting of two parts.[11] One is a chlorotoxin, a protein that can attach itself to chloride channels on a cancer cell surface. The other is a dye that fluoresces when you shine a light on it. So if you inject the paint into a cancer patient's bloodstream, it will attach itself to the tumor. This means the tumor can be made to glow during surgery, making it easier for the surgeon to find and remove. It also makes less invasive surgery possible.

A Paradigm Shift Is Needed

A paradigm shift in the cancer field is needed based upon two fundamental principles of medical practice: 1) do no harm (chemotherapy destroys normal cells and suppresses the immune system with debilitating side effects) and 2) base research and treatment on diseases not on their symptoms or signs. Cancer cells are signs of an underlying disease: neoplasia. The variety of factors in cells and their microenvironments that induce and that fail to block neoplasia in organ systems and tissues should be the focus of research and treatment.

Conclusion

The commonly accepted definition of cancer is responsible for much of the failure of the War on Cancer. We have been intervening after the horse has left the barn.

Words we use determine our perceptions and our actions. So simply fighting cancer by killing cancer cells is not enough and is gravely misleading. If the War on Cancer organized in the late 1930s had become a War on Neoplasia when the latter was clearly identified as the process that produces cancer cells in the 1970s and 1980s, we may well have had effective treatments for the many forms of cancer today.

Unfortunately, a number of potentially significant leads in discovering new approaches to cancer have not been followed because they have not corresponded to established categories and methods of cancer research.

Although proposed in 1957 and subsequent decades, only recently has the focus of cancer research been shifting to why there is a lapse in our bodies' natural defenses in our immune systems that ordinarily detect and destroy abnormal cells that do not die after a normal life span. That lapse permits cancer cells to from through neoplasia and spread.

OLD MODEL: Treatment is determined by a tumor's location in the body without regard for the molecular characteristics of the patient or the tumor and for the microenvironment of the tumor.

NEW MODEL: Research will focus on how cancer cells evade the body's natural defenses in the immune system in the cells' microenvironments. This kind of research is finally beginning to lead to the successful treatment of some forms of cancer and should be given the highest priority. What's more, scientists across disciplines will collaborate on developing innovative cancer treatment and prevention strategies.

We are on the verge of a sea change in how we view and treat cancer. Immunotherapy is leading the way.

Immunotherapy: Drawing upon Your Body's Resources

The ways in which the immune system has been successfully strengthened in the treatment of some cancers and can be expanded to others are noted.

This chapter has two sections. The first explains how important your immune system is to you and how it works. It is worth reading carefully now. The second section is written as a resource for readers with an interest in immunotherapy and its specific forms now or later.

In contrast with traditional surgery, radiation and chemotherapy that aim to kill cancer cells by interventions from outside your body, immunotherapy aims to aid your own body's immune system do its work more efficiently and effectively in stopping neoplasia from producing cancer cells and in removing cancer cells already formed.

Your Immune System

Your immune and nervous systems are similar. Both are dispersed through most of the tissues of your body. Altogether your immune system weighs about 2 pounds. It includes trillions of white blood cells that unlike nervous system cells move about your body freely and about 100 million trillion molecules called antibodies that are produced by your lymphocytes. The special capability of your immune system is pattern recognition; its assignment is to patrol your body and guard its integrity. Immune system cells reach your body tissues through your blood stream and return there through their own lymphatic system which connects your lymph nodes and ultimately returns them to your blood stream. Both your nervous and lymphatic systems build up memories that enable you to adapt to the outside world. Unlike your nervous system, your lymphatic system is subject to continuous decay and renewal.

Your immune system is a complicated web of molecules, cells, tissues and organs that keep your body free of disease, including keeping neoplasia in check. It protects you from millions of bacteria, microbes, viruses, toxins and parasites that would love to invade your body. Some components directly attack bacteria, viruses and aberrant cells. Others gather information for planning an attack and communicate with other cells to carry it out. They all keep you healthy most of the time, but every so often they fail to do their job, and you become ill from infections or from neoplasia. The fact that your immune system plays a key role in preventing the production of cancer cells has been known for a long time.

The moment your immune system stops working the door to your body is wide open. For example, when you die it doesn't take long for organisms to completely dismantle your body so that ultimately all that's left is a skeleton. Your immune system is keeping all of that from happening every minute you are alive. Your immune system is your life line.

The Innate and Adaptive Parts of Your Immune System

Your immune system has two parts: *innate* and *adaptive*. First of all, physical barriers, such as your skin, prevent bacteria and viruses from entering your body. If these invaders breach these barriers, your innate immune system provides an immediate, but non-specific, response that is not lasting.

The major functions of your *innate immune system* include:

+ Recruiting immune cells, such as Natural Killer T Cells, to sites of infection by producing specialized chemicals, such as cytokines.

- Activating immune cells to identify and kill invaders and to clear out dead cells and their products and foreign substances from your organs, tissues, blood stream and lymphatic system.

White blood cells other than lymphocytes play the main role in your innate immune responses. They carry out the many tasks required to protect your body generally against disease-causing microbes and abnormal cells. Some patrol your body seeking foreign invaders and aberrant or dead cells.

If invading cells (pathogens) successfully evade your innate response, a second layer of protection—your *adaptive immune system*—is activated by your innate response. The major functions of your adaptive immune system include:

- Recognizing specific "non-self" characteristics of invading pathogens and of your misbehaving cells.
- Generating specific responses tailored to eliminate pathogens and your aberrant cells.
- Developing immunological memory, in which each pathogen or aberrant cell is "remembered" by immune cell receptors. The memory of these cells can be activated to quickly eliminate that pathogen or aberrant cell type if it subsequently reappears. This is the way immunization works.

White cells, known as lymphocytes, carry out your adaptive immune responses. The most important are B cells and Natural Killer T Cells. B cells make antibodies that bind to, inactivate and help destroy foreign invaders and aberrant cells. Natural Killer T Cells kill infected or aberrant cells by releasing chemicals toxic for them or by prompting the cells to self-destruct. Regulatory T cells can turn these immune cells on and off.

How Your Immune System Works to Prevent and Stop Neoplasia

Normal cells in your body are carefully regulated so that they can perform their functions. Some, such as in moles, do not grow up normally in harmony with their environments and are called dysplastic. They cannot function normally but are tolerated by your immune system because, although they are abnormal, they are not out of control. If they progress into the process of neoplasia, they are regarded as out-of-order aberrant cells and destroyed by your immune system. When dysplastic cells go out of control through neoplasia and are unchecked, they become cancer cells, such as moles turning into melanomas.

Your immune system is blocking neoplasia and preventing cancer cells from growing in your body right now in the same way it deals with bacteria and viruses from outside your body. It has two basic ways of dealing with your own body's misbehaving cells. One involves the release of antibodies from B-cells that lock on to your aberrant cells and trigger

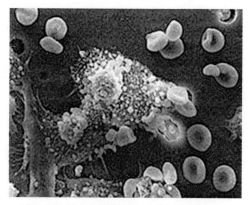

Killer T Cells (smaller white cells) have identified a cancer cell (the large, spiky mass) and are injecting toxins that kill the tumor cell.

other immune cells to come in and sweep them away. In the other, your Natural Killer T Cells seek out and destroy them.

Decades of investigation have made it clear that the interplay between the immune system and cancer is complex. Both the innate and adaptive arms of your immune system discriminate between your normal cells and aberrant cells and can protect you from cancer. Molecules on the surface of your aberrant cells, and perhaps in their interiors, are recognized as different from normal cells by your immune system and thus generate a response to stop your aberrant cells from entering neoplasia, the process that produces cancer cells. Natural Killer T Cells can destroy aberrant cells directly, while B-cells recruit other white cells to do the killing.

Paradoxically your own immune system can facilitate cancer cell development and progression. Elements that normally regulate your immune responses, such as Suppressor Regulatory T Cells, can be stimulated by aberrant cells. This leads to a deficient immune response that is unable to stop the neoplastic growth of cancer cells. In this way, your immune system acts against itself as the microenvironment around the cells suppresses your immune system, permitting dysplastic cells to grow through neoplasia to become cancer cells. Once they emerge from neoplasia, cancer cells have many clever ways to suppress and evade your immune system.

The History of Immunotherapy

In *A Commotion in the Blood* published in 1998, Stephen Hall described how William Coley inoculated cancer patients in the 1890s, first with extracts from human streptococcal abscesses (called "laudable pus") and later with pure cultures of the microbes in order to generally stimulate the immune system and destroy the cancer cells.[1] He claimed successes, but the medical establishment did not embrace his approach because his results could not be reliably reproduced.

Coley's work was supported financially by John D. Rockefeller, Jr., but Rockefeller also supported James Ewing's research on radiation. While Coley told stories of miraculous recoveries, Ewing presented evidence that consistently demonstrated the power of radiation. Ultimately, Rockefeller chose Ewing as his scientific adviser. Rockefeller's support led to the creation of what is now the Memorial Sloan-Kettering Cancer Center. The idea that the body's immune system could play a crucial role in eradicating cancer was largely discarded. One doctor at the time called Coley's hypothesis "whispers of nature."

Still in 1909, the German physician and scientist Paul Ehrlich initiated a century of contentious debate over the immunologic control of neoplasia by proposing that the immune system suppressed the growth of cancer cells. In 1957, the Australian oncologist Frank Burnet expressed the belief that the immune system protects us from developing primary non-viral cancers.[2] In 1963, Dr. Joseph Burchenal of the Memorial Sloan-Kettering Institute for Cancer Research said that "It is unlikely that chemotherapeutic agents against cancer will be any more effective, unless there is some sort of an active immunological response that can be evoked."[3] He pointed out that antibiotics reduce the number of bacteria, but our immune systems are needed to cure the diseases they cause. If the immune system is compromised, such as by AIDS, the patient dies. The same principle applies to chemotherapy and cancer cells.

In 1982, Lewis Thomas presented an overview of the way the immune system works by defining *immunoediting* as a process in which aberrant cells develop mechanisms to permit their multiplication with three possible outcomes:[4]

- Elimination: immunosurveillance distinguishes between aberrant and normal cells and eradicates a significant percentage of the aberrant cells.
- Equilibrium: some aberrant cells withstand the pressure exerted by immunosurveillance's arsenal and may be either killed at the same rate as a tumor grows or permitted to remain as dysplastic benign tumors by immune avoidance mechanisms.

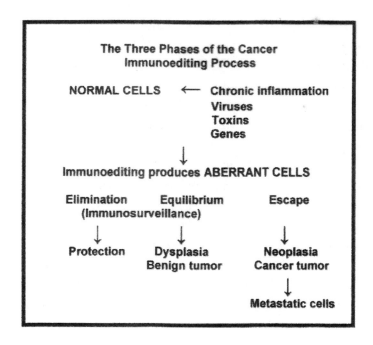

◆   Escape: aberrant tumor cells grow unrestrained by immunosurveillance in the neoplastic process and become cancer cells. In
this way normal cells subject to carcinogenic stimuli ultimately
undergo transformation through neoplasia and become cancer
cells.

Clifton Leaf interviewed Jim Allison, the director of the Tumor-
immunology Program at the Memorial Sloan-Kettering Cancer Center,
who began his career as a researcher at the University of Texas Cancer
Center in 1978.[5] At that time, he was taken with the idea that cancer cells
can disarm the immune system by producing proteins that cause Natural
Killer T Cells (NKTC) to either quickly become exhausted and die or
blithely overlook the tumor. Allison's research focused on why NKTC
failed to recognize cancer cells as being aberrant and attack them, as they
do with bacteria and viruses.

Allison's mentors discouraged him from pursuing research on
NKTC. "Tumor immunology had such a bad reputation many people
thought that the immune system didn't play any role in cancer," he said.
But Allison started looking at how the immune system fights disease in
mice models and capitalized on a critical discovery: NKTC require two
signals to attack a target effectively. The first signal is "like the ignition
switch" and the second is "like the gas pedal". Signal one enables the
NKTC to recognize a component of a cancer cell as its target. Signal
two tells the NKTC what to do. When working against a microbe, both
signals operate. But, in the presence of cancer cells the "ignition switch"
signal can either turn the cell on or off. If the signal is turned on, the
NKTC become activated and proliferate throughout the body, seeking
out and destroying cancer cells. If the signal is turned off, the NKTC do
not respond.

The American Cancer Society vindicated Allison in 2012 by noting that better understanding of the biology of cancer cells has led to
developing biologic agents that mimic some of the natural signals the
body uses to control cell activity and growth. Clinical trials have shown
that this cancer treatment—called biological response modifier therapy,

biologic therapy, biotherapy or immunotherapy—is enduringly effective for several cancers. It focuses on neoplasia.

Still, strengthening the immune system's role in eliminating cancer cells proposed repeatedly since 1957 started being taken seriously only recently as the focus of research and treatment. Researchers have been distracted by the allure and excitement generated by expanding knowledge about the human genome. They have not paid sufficient attention to the facts that 1) the functions of genes are controlled by factors in the cellular environment (epigenetically) that enhance or suppress the growth of cancer cells and that 2) the genes in cancer cells change rapidly as they mutate.

The last fifteen years have seen a re-emergence and an enhanced understanding of Burchenal and Thomas's observations. Some scientists have been successfully studying immunoediting and immunosurveillance as counterpoints to the dominant "search for and destroy cancer cells" model. They are finding ways to help the immune system do its job through immunotherapy that prevents and stops neoplasia.

A 2004 article in the journal *Immunity* summarized the work on the cancer immunoediting and immunosurveillance processes—underscoring hope that an enhanced understanding of naturally occurring immune system/tumor interactions will lead to the development of more effective immunologically based cancer therapies.[6] In support of this trend, Michael Sporn, professor of pharmacology and medicine at Dartmouth Medical School, advocates preventing carcenogenesis—neoplasia—from entering the deadly stage of cancer cells in the first place.[7]

The interaction between the immune system, prostate cancer and melanoma has been an area of research interest for several decades. The recent Food and Drug Administration approval of two immunotherapies (prostate: sipuleucel-T and melanoma: ipilimumab) has stimulated broader interest in using the immune system to fight neoplasia and in developing predictive biomarkers for selecting patients for combinations of these treatments and for providing building blocks for future immunotherapies.[8]

After decades of neglect, immunotherapy finally was recognized appropriately at the 2013 American Association for Cancer Research (AACR) meeting. In her plenary lecture, Dr. Suzanne Topalian of Johns Hopkins University said that despite the current dogma that cancer is a genetic disease, it also can be viewed as an immunologic disorder.[9] She said, "In many ways the adaptive immune system is an ideal anti-cancer therapy." She affirmed in 2013 a concept first advanced in 1957 by Dr. Frank Burnet and reiterated in the 1980s and 1990s. The 2014 AACR annual meeting focused on the most recent progress in cancer genomics that supports the notion that cancer is immunogenic. The dynamic interplay among malignant cells, immune cells and the immunosuppressive tumor microenvironment leads to the escape of tumors from host immune surveillance. Long-term survival benefits were reported in several cancer types as the potential of cancer immunotherapies is just starting to be realized.

It is not an understatement to say that immunotherapy is a major change in cancer treatment. Cancer in the past has been largely treated by surgery, chemotherapy and/or radiation. All pose the challenge of sparing healthy tissue from irreparable damage while ensuring that every cancer cell is destroyed. This new trend is supported by the Federation of Clinical Immunology Societies, an organization devoted to improving human health through immunology by fostering interdisciplinary approaches to understand and treat immune-based diseases, including cancer.

Immunotherapies

This section summarizes the concepts and technologies of the various forms of immunotherapy.

The aim of immunotherapy is to stimulate the immune system to prevent or stop neoplasia. This can be done either by activating the immune system to destroy cancer cells while avoiding stimulating immune system suppressor elements or by training the immune system to recognize cancer cells as targets to be destroyed. There are four categories of immunotherapy: active, adoptive, restorative and passive.

Active Immunotherapy

Active immunotherapy aims to stimulate a patient's innate immune response to neoplasia, either nonspecifically or specifically.

Nonspecific active immunotherapy uses agents that stimulate immune system activity in general. Certain cytokines, such as interferons and interleukins, have been used to stimulate an immune system response against cancer cells. Because the direct administration of such cytokines may cause systemic inflammation resulting in serious side effects, a new generation of chimeric cytokine molecules that can be made in laboratories has been developed to provide an effective yet localized immune response that destroys the cancer cells without unwanted side-effects. An infamous case of something going disastrously wrong with immunotherapy was a clinical trial in 2006 at Northwick Park Hospital in London where scientists were testing a powerful immunotherapeutic drug on six volunteers. All suffered serious side effects caused by the overstimulation of their immune systems.[10] This emphasizes the fact that the immune system can work against the body as it does in autoimmune disorders.

Interferon alpha is approved for the treatment of some cancers, including melanoma and chronic myeloid leukemia, and is being studied for use with other cancers. An interferon IL-2 is approved as an anti-cancer treatment, particularly for kidney cancers and melanomas that have metastasized to other regions of the body.

Currently, bacillus Calmette-Guérin (BCG) is the only immunotherapy agent approved by the Food and Drug Administration as the primary therapy of carcinoma in situ of the bladder. It stimulates an inflammatory immune response in the bladder wall that destroys cancer cells. Typically, BCG is administered weekly for 6 weeks. Periodic follow-up usually is necessary to assess its long-term effectiveness. It is most often used after cancer has been removed from the bladder using transurethral resection surgery.[11]

Specific active immunotherapy stimulates the immune system to target particular proteins called antigens on cancer cells. One form of specific active immunotherapy involves activating immune cells by removing them from the body and enriching them with cytokines in the laboratory. Specificity is attained by exposing these white blood cells to a particular antigen associated with a specific cancer. This exposure "trains" the white blood cells to target and destroy the cancer cells when they are transfused back into the patient.

In 2010, the FDA approved Sipuleucel-T (Provenge), a cancer vaccine for prostate cancer that has spread and is no longer responding to hormone treatment. Provenge is made by culturing a patient's own immune cells with an antigen that is prostate cancer specific. When infused into the patient, the vaccine activates Natural Killer T Cells to target and attack prostate cancer cells. This treatment has been shown to help certain men with prostate cancer live longer, though it does not cure their diseases.

Cancer vaccines have limitations because they are targeted. Not all cancer cell antigens are the same, and the cells with their antigens mutate. They also mutate as a result of chemotherapy and radiation treatment. If the target changes, the vaccines become ineffective. Infusing back into a cancer patient cells that have been modified in a laboratory also is not completely without risk and may be associated with immediate and delayed hypersensitivity reactions that can be life threatening.

Adoptive immunotherapy

Vaccines attempt to get the body's immune system cells to respond more effectively by exposing them to specific cancer antigens. In contrast, adoptive immunotherapy involves removing immune system cells from a patient, boosting their anti-cancer activity by genetically recoding them to identify and seek out proteins present on cancer cells, growing them in large numbers and then returning them to the patient.

Novartis is studying chimeric antigen receptor (CAR T) technology in which Natural Killer T Cells (NKTC) are extracted from the patient's blood.[12] These cells are genetically re-coded. This enables chimeric antigen receptors (CARs) on NKTC to recognize specific cancer cell antigens that they would otherwise view as harmless in order to promote killing the cancer cells. Scientists at the National Institutes of Health have developed CARs with high affinity for the ErbB2 antigen, which is overexpressed in a variety of cancer cells, including lung, breast, colorectal, ovary, prostate and head and neck squamous cell cancers. These ErbB2-specific CARs on NKTC (CAR T) could prove to be powerful new immunotherapeutic tools for attacking ErbB2 cancer cells.

At the 2013 American Association for Cancer Research (AACR) meeting, Renier Brentjens of the Memorial Sloan-Kettering Cancer Center in New York reported early-stage clinical successes in acute lymphocytic leukemia (ALL) with the use of chimeric antigen receptor T (CAR T) cells.[13] Other researchers reported similarly encouraging results with CAR T-cell therapy used to treated children with relapsed ALL. Brentjens described these as "armored" CAR T cells that can not only kill, but also "insert a factory into the tumor" to produce molecules that protect the immune cells from a hostile microenvironment. In one study, all 5 adults and 19 of 22 children with ALL had a complete remission, meaning no cancer could be found after treatment, although a few have relapsed since then. These were gravely ill patients out of options. Some had tried multiple bone marrow transplants and up to 10 types of chemotherapy or other treatments.

At the 2014 AACR meeting, Carl June of the Abramson Cancer Center at the University of Pennsylvania said that researchers are now working out which genes can be inserted into NKTC to further promote target specificity, potency and persistence.[14] He also cautioned that CAR T cell therapy requires researchers to tailor genetically modified cells to individual patients, so it is not currently practical for large-scale application.

Researchers in Japan have shown for the first time that it is possible to make cancer-specific immune system cells from stem cells that have the potential to become any kind of cell.[15] Their work brings closer the day when therapies use cloned versions of patients' own cells to boost their immune systems' natural ability to kill cancer cells.

Researchers at the University of Georgia are developing a new technique that uses nanoparticles to reprogram immune cells so they are able to recognize and attack cancer cells. If the nanoparticle process becomes a treatment, doctors could biopsy a tumor from the patient and kill the cancer cells with nanoparticles. They could then produce dendritic cells activated by the killed cancer cells in bulk quantities in the laboratory and inject them into a patient. Once in the bloodstream, the newly activated cells would alert the immune system to the cancer cells' presence to destroy them. Researcher Shanta Dhar said, "for the first time we can stimulate the immune system to act against breast cancer cells through mitochondria-targeted nanoparticles… using a novel pathway."[16]

Restorative Immunotherapy

Restorative immunotherapy is the direct and indirect restoration of deficient functions of immune system cells through any means other than removing them from a patient. Examples are *reactivating NKTC, unblocking NKTC proliferation* and *NKTC Receptor Bispecific Therapy.*

After they have been activated, NKTC begin to produce the molecule PD-1 on their surfaces. This turns them off in order to keep the immune response from over-reacting.[17] Even if the NKTC can recognize a cancer tumor and can get to the tumor, once it gets there and the cancer cells produce PD-L-1—a partner molecule to PD-1—the NKTC's anti-cancer activity will be turned off. As an immunotherapy, an anti-PD-1 antibody can be used to block PD-1 and PD-L-1 and *reactivate NKTC* by turning their anti-cancer activity back on.

In recent clinical trials, anti–PD-1 antibody treatment has led to favorable responses in patients with several types of advanced metastatic cancer, but only a minority of these patients derived long-term benefit from this treatment. The fact that a combination of IL-2 and anti-PD-1 antibodies has been used clinically in cancer patients makes research with them well worth pursuing and suggests one way in which the impressive results seen in some patients may be extended to more patients with currently untreatable disease.[18]

Ipilimumab is a monoclonal antibody made by Bristol-Myers-Squib that recognizes and binds to a molecule called CTLA-4, another immune response suppressor found on NKTC.[19] CTLA-4 normally keeps NKTC from proliferating, but in the presence of ipilimumab, it is blocked, allowing NKTC to increase in numbers so that they can attack cancer cells. Ipilimumab works by *unblocking the NKTC proliferation* blocking effect of CTLA-4.

For the past 20 years, the former academics who set up the company Immunocore have worked on realizing their dream of developing a totally new approach to cancer treatment called *Natural Killer T-cell Receptor Bispecific Therapy* by harnessing the power of the immune system's NKTC.[20]

Immunocore has found a way of designing small protein molecules, which it calls ImmTACs, that effectively act as double-ended glue. At one end they stick to cancer cells, strongly and very specifically, leaving healthy cells untouched. At the other end they stick to NKTC. This technology is based on the NKTC receptor protein that sticks out of the surface of the Natural Killer T Cell and binds to its enemy target. Immunocore's ImmTACs bind strongly to cancer cells at one end and to NKTC at the other end—thus bringing cancer cells to their nemesis. This forces NKTC to recognize cancer cells, suggesting that it can be used in any kind of cancer.

The key to the success of the technique is being able to distinguish between a cancer cell and a normal, healthy cell. Immunocore's drug does this by recognizing small proteins or peptides that stick out from the surface membrane of cancer cells. These peptides act like a shop window, revealing what is going on within the cell and whether or not it is cancer.

Immunocore is building up a database of peptide targets on cancer cells in order to hopefully design NKTC receptors that can target them, leaving healthy cells alone and so minimizing possible side effects.

A risk with deploying NKTC against cancer is their potency. Yet this very potency is exciting because it could lead to treatment for metastatic disease that has spread throughout the body.

Passive Immunotherapy

Passive immunotherapy is infusing a patient with antibodies to antigens on the patient's cancer cells and thereby destroying the cells.

Examples are *monoclonal antibodies, Epithelial Mesenchymal Transition Therapy, Transient Photoactivation and Laser Assisted Immunotherapy,* block the *"don't-eat-me"* signal and *training the immune system to attack the tumor.*

Monoclonal antibodies are laboratory-made versions of immune system proteins. Antibodies can be useful in treating neoplasia because they can be designed to attack a specific part of a cancer cell. Using technology that was first developed during the 1970s, scientists can mass-produce monoclonal antibodies that are specifically targeted to chemical components of cancer cells.[21] Refinements to these methods, using recombinant DNA technology, have improved the effectiveness and decreased the side effects of these treatments. The first therapeutic monoclonal antibodies—rituximab (Rituxan) and trastuzumab (Herceptin)—were approved during the late 1990s to treat lymphoma and HER2-positive breast cancer respectively. Monoclonal antibodies now are used to treat a growing number of cancers.

Scientists from the Manchester Collaborative Center for Inflammation Research discovered that rituximab—a chimeric monoclonal antibody—tended to stick to one side of the cancer cell, forming a cap and drawing a number of proteins over to that side. It effectively created a front and back to the cell—with a cluster of protein molecules massed on one side. What surprised the scientists the most was how this changed the effectiveness of NKTC in destroying these diseased cells. When the NKTC approached, they stood an 80 percent chance of killing the cancer cell if they latched on to the side where the protein was collected. In contrast, when the cancer cell lacked this cluster of proteins on one side, it was killed only 40 percent of the time.[22] Rituximab is an effective drug because it identifies cancer cells and signals cells of the immune system to come in and sweep the cancer cells away.

Scientists from the University of California-San Diego School of Medicine have identified a protein ROR1 that seems to serve as a switch, regulating the spread of cancer cells from the primary tumor to distant spots in the body.[23] The protein is used by embryo cells during early development in a process known as *epithelial mesenchymal transition* (EMT) but disappears from the body after a baby is born. Through the EMT process, embryonic cells migrate and eventually grow into tissues and organs in the fetus.

According to the researchers, ROR1 was only found in people with metastatic cancer, leading them to believe that regulating this protein might stop the metastasis. The lead investigator Dr. Thomas Kipps said, "The protein seems to get turned off after embryonic development, and we've only identified a small sub-population of cells that can turn it on."[24]

ROR1's role during embryonic development may explain how it helps cancers to grow and spread in adult life. It's a protein that sits on the surface of the cancer cell. Half of it sits outside the cell and half inside the cell. It's like having an antenna sticking out with a transmitter below the surface. That transmitter conveys important signals to the cell, and it seems to encourage cancer cells to migrate.

In a series of lab experiments, Kipps and his team found that high-level expression of ROR1 in breast cancer cells were associated with higher rates of relapse and metastasis. However, when they used therapies to silence the expression of ROR1, the researchers were able to inhibit metastatic spread of the cancer cells in animal models. It's like taking the antenna away; you can't hear the radio or TV station anymore. The cancer cells become more fragile and don't grow as well. Since ROR1 is only expressed in cancer cells, Kipps said, "it provides a singular target for future therapies aimed at containing and reversing metastasis. Then, once the cancer becomes more localized, traditional therapies such as radiation and surgery can help remove the original tumor from the body."

In a process called *Transient Photoactivation* Cardiff University researchers have created a peptide (a small piece of protein) linked to a light-responsive dye that can switch "on" death pathways in B-cell lymphoma cancer cells. The peptide remains inactive until exposed to external light pulses, which convert it into a cell death signal in a "smart" and controlled way. This new pathway activation technology may enable scientists to develop more effective treatment strategies.[25]

Laser-Assisted Immunotherapy uses a precise laser beam to destroy the primary tumor sensitized by a chemical that makes cancer cells more vulnerable to destruction by the laser without unacceptably heating nearby normal cells, and then delivers a powerful boost to the immune system's natural cancer defense systems. In this way, the entire immune system joins the fight against an individual's own specific cancer.[26]

At the 2014 meeting of the American Association of Cancer Research, scientists at the Stanford School of Medicine noted that nearly all cancers use the molecule CD47 as a "don't-eat-me" signal to escape from being eaten and eliminated by macrophages.[27] The researchers found that anti-CD47 antibodies, which can *block the "don't-eat-me" signal* and enable macrophages to engulf cancer cells, eliminated or inhibited the growth of various blood cancers and solid tumors. The Stanford group plans to start human clinical trials of the anti-CD47 cancer therapy.

According to Dr. Clifford A. Hudis, chief of breast cancer medicine service at Memorial Sloan Kettering Cancer Center in New York, scientists are now developing techniques to outsmart the cancer cell's aggressive tactics by prompting the patient's immune system to launch a continuous attack that keeps the disease at bay indefinitely.[28] An approach under study involves destroying the tumor by freezing it with an ice probe, but leaving it in place in the body and thus *training the immune system to attack to attack the tumor*. The patient then is given an immune stimulant to help overcome the molecular obstacles that had kept the immune system from recognizing the cancer as foreign tissue.

Tumor Microenvironment

It's clear now that a focus on cancer cells is only part of the problem in neoplasia. The diverse mass of non-malignant cells surrounding, supporting and infiltrating a tumor that comprise the tumor microenvironment (TME) also plays a key role in the progression of disease.[29] "It's not a single rogue cell; it takes a village of cells," said Mina Bissell, a cell biologist at the Lawrence Berkeley National Laboratory in California, in a 2013 AACR session on how interactions between malignant and non-malignant cells influence cancer growth and on how the molecular pathways of communication can be targeted.

Dr. Susan Love of the Dr. Susan Love Research Foundation is excited about the prospect of fighting or preventing cancer by changing the "microenvironment" of the breast—the tissue surrounding a tumor that can stimulate or halt its growth.[30] She likened it to the way living in a good or bad neighborhood might sway a potentially delinquent child. "It may well be that by altering the 'neighborhood,' whether it's the immune system or the local tissue, we can control or kill the cancer cells." Taking hormone-replacement therapy during menopause, which was found to contribute to escalating rates of breast cancer, may have been the biological equivalent of letting meth dealers colonize a street corner. On the other hand, immunotherapy would be like putting more cops on the beat.

Androgen Deprivation Therapy (ADT), a mainstay of treatment for both high-risk early prostate cancer and recurrent and/or metastatic disease, has been shown to positively alter the immune environment in prostate cancer.[31] For example, ADT with prostate cancer patients results in increased numbers of immune system cells in prostate tissues.

Frances Balkwill of Barts Cancer Institute in London presented her work at the 2013 AACR meeting on certain ovarian cancers.[32] Using mouse transplant models, Balkwill demonstrated that up to fifty percent of primary and metastatic tumor masses is comprised of CD4+, CD8+ macrophages, B cells and fibroblasts surrounding the tumor itself. Balkwill said that these cells together with inflammatory cytokines including interleukin-6 (IL-6) appear to be responsible for facilitating the growth and spread of tumors. (An example of how the immune system can work against itself.) She also presented clinical data showing that an anti-IL-6 antibody results in rapid reduction of inflammation and tumor mass and so may open a window of opportunity for immunotherapy. There are enough commonalities to suggest that targeting non-malignant cells and the molecules that mediate their communication with the tumors they surround should have applications across different cancers.

Also at the 2013 AACR meeting, Shahin Rafii of Cornell University Medical College discussed how growth factors secreted by endothelial cells in the blood vessels and around tumors—known as angiogenic factors—support cancer cell progression.[33] "Crosstalk between cancer cells and blood vessel endothelial cells promotes the generation of a vasculature that fosters expansion of chemo-resistant, tumor-initiating cells," he said. Rafii also presented data showing that targeting a protein called Jagged-1 in the endothelial cells of blood vessels may be sufficient to increase chemotherapy sensitivity and slow tumor growth in certain cancers.

At the same AACR meeting, Larry Norton, an oncologist at the Memorial Sloan-Kettering Cancer Center, said that "the field is starting to come together to build a comprehensive picture" of the tumor micro-environment. He also argued that the emerging concepts of how the TME influences tumor cell behavior could help make sense of the flood of genomic data relating to the initiation and growth of cancer.[34]

A gene in the TME has been discovered that stops the spread of cancer cells. To metastasize, cancer cells must override sticky molecular anchors protruding from the cell membrane that typically keep the cells rooted within their respective locations. Deviously, cancer cells can switch these anchors off, allowing them to traverse the body through the bloodstream and take up residence in new organs. About a fifth of lung cancer cases are missing an anti-cancer gene called LKB1 and are often aggressive, rapidly spreading through the body. LKB1 is in the microenvironment of cells as a part of the immune system. In 2014 a Salk Institute for Biological Studies team reported the discovery of a little-known gene called DIXDC1 that receives instructions from LKB1 to activate the molecular anchor cells.[35] Tumors have two ways to turn off this "stay-put" signal and enable cells to break away from a tumor and travel through the bloodstream and dock at organs throughout the body. One is by inhibiting DIXDC1 directly. The other way is by deleting LKB1, which then never sends the signal to DIXDC1 to "turn on" the focal adhesions to anchor the cell. This discovery may lead to ways to block tumor cells from turning off the "stay put" signal.

The Tumor Microenvironment Initiative of the National Cancer Institute (NCI) focuses on expanding understanding of the role of the TME in cancer initiation, progression and metastasis. Through this initiative, the National Cancer Institute Division of Cancer Biology intends to generate a more comprehensive understanding of the composition of the microenvironment in normal tissues with the goal of delineating the mechanisms of tumor microenvironmental interactions in human cancer.

Eleven funded centers form the Tumor Microenvironment Network (TMEN), an infrastructure intended to promote and facilitate interdisciplinary collaboration and progress in understanding the role of the microenvironment in neoplasia.[36] In addition, TMEN has ten Collaborative U01 programs that bring together a TMEN key investigator and scientists with expertise in other biological systems or organ sites not currently being studied within TMEN to form a new project in tumor microenvironment research.

Autoimmune Therapy

Autoimmune diseases that have devastating consequences for healthy tissue are prime examples of how your immune system can work against your body's interests. This explains why it has essential ways of regulating itself that can backfire in its mission to destroy aberrant cells.

In mice, the same cells that can drive the body to destroy its own tissue have been used to destroy cancer cells. A recently discovered type of immune cell called Th17 plays a key role in autoimmune disease in which the immune system mistakenly identifies the body's own tissues as foreign and attacks them.[37] Natalia Martin-Orozco believes that Th17 cells recognize cancer cells and, in response, release chemicals that attract immune cells called dendritic cells to the cancer cells. These cells seize tumor proteins and take them to lymph nodes where Natural Killer T Cells recognize and attack them.[38]

An interesting sidelight about autoimmune diseases is that bacteria actually can protect us from autoimmune diseases if we grew up with them early in life, even while in our mothers' wombs. Naturally occurring bacteria found on farms, for example, stimulate the growth of Regulatory T cells that are at low levels in autoimmune diseases, like asthma and allergies. Amish farmers are examples of people who are less prone to allergies than most Americans.[39]

Society for Immunotherapy of Cancer

Founded in 1984, the Society for Immunotherapy of Cancer (SITC) is an organization of clinicians, researchers, students, post-doctoral fellows and allied health professionals dedicated to improving cancer patient outcomes by advancing the development and application of cancer immunotherapy.

The 28th annual meeting of the SITC was held on November 7-10, 2013. The topics covered at this meeting included advances in cancer treatment using adoptive cell therapy, oncolytic viruses, dendritic cells, immune check point modulators and combination therapies. Advances in immune editing of cancer, immune modulation by cancer and the tumor microenvironment also were discussed.

SITC launched the *Journal for ImmunoTherapy of Cancer* in 2012. The new journal encompasses all aspects of tumor immunology and cancer immunotherapy from basic research to clinical application. Today, more than ever before, excitement in the field and increased momentum brought about by the latest approvals of immunotherapy-based treatments in various forms of cancer have shown the clear need for the *Journal*.[40]

DNA Sequencing in the Mutanome

Genetic changes in the mass of a person's cancer cells (the mutanome) encode unique m-peptides that can be targets for Natural Killer T Cells. Recent advances in next-generation sequencing and computation prediction allow, for the first time, the rapid and affordable identification of m-peptides in individual patients.[41] Inexpensive and highly available DNA sequencing may revolutionize cancer immunotherapy by enabling highly personalized approaches involving the identification of new tumor-associated antigens.

The Federal Drug Administration

Immunology and immunotherapy are experiencing increased momentum, catalyzed by the latest approvals of immunotherapy-based treatments in multiple cancer types. More cancer vaccine candidates, monoclonal antibodies and cellular therapies are showing promise, and major pharmaceutical companies are driving their development into novel cancer treatments. They see that immunotherapy is the missing link in cancer treatment that possibly can give lasting remissions.

A picture of what the Federal Drug Administration (FDA) is looking for in cancer immunotherapy product development appears in an extensive review article published in the inaugural issue of the *Journal for ImmunoTherapy of Cancer*.[42] Written by members of the FDA's Office of Cellular, Tissue and Gene Therapies, this review provides a regulatory perspective on pre-clinical to first-in-human studies. It's particularly timely as the field of cancer immunotherapy is quickly advancing especially now after promising new data was released from several early phase clinical trials showing significant tumor shrinkage and long-term durable response rates in cancer patients treated with various new cancer immunotherapies, such as Genentech's MPDL3280A and Bristol-Myers Squibb's nivolumab. More positive data including the use of combination treatments like ipilimumab (Yervoy) with nivolumab also show significant tumor shrinkage in patients with melanoma when used together rather than by themselves.

The FDA review addressed the previous policy of only using immunotherapy treatment in advanced and metastatic disease patients. It's now understood that both early and late stage patients can be included in immunotherapy trials, and considerations for both settings are being addressed. The importance of keeping patients who show signs of early tumor progression on a study from which they may benefit later also was discussed.

By 2013, thirteen immunotherapy antibodies had been approved by the FDA and many more are currently being evaluated in clinical trials.[43] Drug companies have an incentive to speed development of immunotherapy drugs. They are expected to be profitable with a great demand.

Because of new data in the field of cancer immunotherapy, this is a crucial time for all involved in the treatment of cancer.

The National Cancer Institute

The National Cancer Institute has an important role in funding cancer centers and projects that support the ongoing treatment of cancer. At the same time, it has an obligation to the public to emphasize research that focuses on enabling the body's natural defenses to do their job in eliminating precancerous and cancer cells resulting from neoplasia and that thereby leads to effective and enduring treatments for cancer. As advocated by American Society of Clinical Oncology, the Institute has a key role to play in fostering the determination of the causes of neoplasia and what can be done about those causes.

Conclusion

The need for accelerating the progress of cancer research and treatment to improve patient care is obvious. There are a variety of factors that induce neoplasia in organ systems and tissues that should be the focus of research and treatment.

While each immunotherapy involves a part of the immune system, available evidence suggests that combination immunotherapy has the potential to most closely resemble the ways in which your natural immune system works. Combining immunotherapies with other treatments in an effort to improve results is beginning to gain traction as well. Moreover, we can imagine scenarios where these approaches are likely to reduce the need for extensive surgery.

So far, immunotherapy drugs have been found to help patients with melanoma, kidney, prostate and lung cancers. In preliminary studies, they also appear to be effective in breast cancer; ovarian cancer and cancers of the colon, stomach, head and neck. Drug companies have an incentive to speed development of immunotherapy drugs. They are expected to be profitable with a great demand for them.

The editor-in-chief of *Science* Marcia McNutt selected immunotherapy as the scientific "Breakthrough of the Year 2013" that marks a significant moment in cancer history and merits recognition and celebration, even if uncertainties remain.

Nutritional Therapy: Drawing on Nature's Resources

The long-delayed application of knowledge about neoplasia as a metabolic disorder that can respond to the foods and supplements we eat is outlined.

The new way to look at cancer...by tracing its deep roots to the dawn of living cells more than a billion years ago... proposed by Paul Davies and Charles Lineweaver may well transform cancer research and treatment.[1] If their theory is correct, it promises to link the origin of cancer to the origin of life and to the development of human embryos. They predict that saturating cancer cells with oxygen and depriving them of sugar will slow them down and even kill them, echoing Otto Warburg who made the same prediction in 1924.

Neoplasia Requires Glucose

Each cell in your body is an exceedingly complicated machine in which all functions are carefully regulated. Your normal cells divide only when they need to do so. A cancer cell divides unnecessarily and too often. This means that a cancer cell's regulators are out of order.

A variety of factors in your body ensure that your cells only grow and divide when appropriate.[2] But cancer cells are different from other cells. Something in their regulation breaks down, and they start growing and dividing rapidly in the process of neoplasia. They start hoarding energy from the blood; then they manipulate their surroundings to support their rapid growth. As previously pointed out, one vital fact about cancer cells is that they rely on much more glucose from the blood as their source of energy than do normal cells.

Otto Warburg came up with the idea that cancer is caused by cells mainly generating energy by the breakdown of glucose without using oxygen (a process called glycolysis) and the subsequent process of fermentation. This is in contrast with healthy cells that mainly generate energy from the breakdown of glucose using oxygen within their mitochondria. The observation that the "Warburg effect", described in Chapter Five, was such a consistent and dominate aspect of cancer led Warburg to propose that abnormal mitochrondrial metabolism is the origin of cancer. He put it this way: "Cancer, above all other diseases, has countless secondary causes. But, even for cancer, there is only one prime cause. Summarized in a few words, the prime cause of cancer is the replacement of the respiration of oxygen in normal body cells by a fermentation of sugar."[3] Warburg set the stage for Davies and Lineweaver's contemporary evolutionary theory.

Energy production with oxygen is far more efficient than fermentation. Almost 20 times more energy is released when glucose is completely oxidized, as opposed to when it is fermented. Oxidative energy production takes place in mitochondria commonly referred to as a cell's "power plants" because their primary function is to supply the body with its energy requirements.

The metabolic theory of cancer contends that it begins with damage to the mitochondria that knocks down oxidative energy production. The cell then is forced to produce energy through fermentation in order to survive. Because a cancer cell's mitochondria are damaged, the cell is forced to generate energy by inefficient fermentation and has to consume much more glucose to live. A glance at a positron emission tomography (PET) scan, which uses a radioactive labeled form of glucose to image cancer tumors, provides visual evidence of the voracious appetite cancer cells have for glucose compared to normal cells...cancer tumors stand out in bold relief against surrounding normal cells.

Albert Szent-Gyorgyi, a Hungarian Nobel Prize Winner, continued the theory that the fundamental cause of cancer is a disturbance in cell metabolism that makes a cell prefer fermentation of glucose for energy production rather than the more efficient oxidative metabolism, which requires oxygen.[4] The fermentation of glucose does occur in normal cell division, but a normal cell reverts back after dividing to oxidative metabolism, which requires an organized cell structure. Therefore, it may be that the uncontrolled growth of cancer cells arises when they are stuck in the fermentation process. This raises questions about what keeps them stuck in that process or what turns off the ability of the cell to revert back to normal oxidative cell metabolism. Both questions point to a defect in cell metabolic regulation.

One of the mysteries about cancer has been that it rarely emerges from muscle cells. This may be because they are so dependent on oxygen and oxidative metabolism or so rich in mitochondria, their power centers, that there is too much oxidative reserve for cancer to develop. Cancer cells can't stand oxygen.

As mentioned before, cancer cells have lost their capacity to conduct oxidation and to use oxygen for useful work. Instead a low-grade process—wasteful fermentation—is used to produce energy. Warburg suggested, but could not prove, that this fermentation was due to "abnormal mitochondria", that is, cancer cells are forced to use inefficient, non-mitochondrial means of generating energy because their mitochondria are not working properly. Szent-Gyorgyi suggested that this fermentation energy forces cell division. In other words, efficient oxidative energy production is associated with an organized cell structure, whereas fermentation is associated with cell disorganization and the resulting inclination to cell division. When cancer cells multiply, they simply are performing the unregulated innate function of cell division that is not controlled. Szent-Gyorgyi believed that this apparent mitochondrial dysfunction is, in fact, reversible.

Mitrochondria—The Glucose Consuming Energy Producers

Mitochondria are the primary sources of energy production in a cell, producing 80% of its energy needs. Several differences have been observed between the mitochondria of cancer cells and those of normal cells suggesting to researchers as long ago as 1945 that mutations in mitochondria might cause cancer.[5] Various cancer cell lines show differences in the number, size and shape of mitochondria compared to normal cells.[6] In addition, the mitochondria of rapidly growing cancer tumors tend to be fewer in number, smaller and have fewer

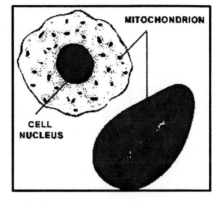

internal folds than the mitochondria of slowly growing tumors. What's more, alterations in the inner membrane composition of cancer cell mitochondria were reported in 2002. Cancer cells also have been shown to have more hyperpolarized mitochondria and to be relatively deficient in potassium channels.[7]

More recently mitochondria also have been found to be integrally involved in apoptosis—programmed cell death.[8] This suggests that mitochondrial dysfunction might block apoptosis and promote unregulated cell division. The mitochondria contain their own DNA (less than 1% of the amount of nuclear DNA), which seems to be more susceptible to damage and mutations than nuclear DNA. So it turns out that mitochondrial dysfunction actually is one of the prominent features of cancer cells. Incidentally, the accumulation of mutations in mitochondrial DNA also is thought to play a causative role in aging.

All the available evidence suggests that, if we want to understand cancer better, we need to turn our attention to mitochondria, for it is here that the energy malfunctions occurring in cancer are found. If they can be reversed, normal cell death (apoptosis) might be increased and neoplastic cancer cell growth prevented.[9]

Dichloroacetate (DCA) significantly increases glucose oxidation in mitochondria, indicating that the metabolic cancer signature of glucose fermentation is reversible, rather than a consequence of permanent mitochondrial damage. In the 1950s, Albert Szent-Gyorgyi concluded this as did William Koch.[10] At the present time, though approved as a drug treatment for mitochondrial diseases in humans and apart from anecdotal reports, there are no formally completed clinical trials of DCA treatment in patients with cancer. There apparently are significant side effects that need to be taken into account.

Further evidence that compromised mitochondrial function is a fundamental cause of neoplasia also is suggested by the reported efficacy of the Kucera Cancer Support Regime, which stresses cruciferous vegetables, such as arugula, bok choy, broccoli, cabbage, cauliflower, collard greens, kale and watercress. Michael Kucera, a Czech physician, spent over 20 years in the late 1990s researching mitochondrial medicine and developed nutritional combinations for supporting mitochondrial health.[11] A combination of these nutrients with immune system support nutrients led to cancer remissions. He reported that over 700 cancer patients (including breast, prostate, colon and gastric cancers), most already metastatic, had been treated with this regime. Overall a 70% remission at 5 years was reported and an 80-90% remission when the formulas were combined with chemotherapy. No side effects were observed. A regime like this is used at the Chiron Clinic in London to treat cancer. The basis for the diet's efficacy may well be due to its benefits for mitochondria.

Paul Talalay, Professor of Pharmacology and Molecular Sciences at Johns Hopkins University, found that cruciferous vegetables reduce and may block neoplasia.[12] He demonstrated in his laboratory that a topical extract of broccoli can protect skin cells against cancer-promoting damage from the sun.

To top off of all of this suggestive evidence, Thomas Seyfried in his 2012 book *Cancer as a Metabolic Disease*, makes a compelling case for the metabolic factors that lead to neoplasia.[13] In this theory, disruption of cellular oxidation precedes and underlies the genetic instability that accompanies cancer development. Once established, genetic instability contributes to further cell oxidative impairment, genetic mutations and cancer progression. In other words, effects become causes in the neoplastic process. This hypothesis is based on evidence that the integrity of the genes in a cell nucleus is largely dependent on normal mitochondrial energy production.

Cigarette smoke, chemicals and other carcinogens damage mitochondrial DNA. Once damaged the mitochondria send out signals that activate a series of important neoplastic pathways, altering huge swaths of "stop" and "go" genes. When taken together they cause uncontrolled neoplasia and further gene instability—the most salient features of cancer.

Two major conclusions emerge from the hypothesis that neoplasia is a metabolic disease: 1) many cancers may regress and 2) many cancers may be prevented if carbohydrate intake is restricted. These conclusions are supported by the fact that obesity is a risk factor for cancer. Consequently, carbohydrate restricted diets combined with agents that reduce glucose may provide a rational strategy for the long-term management and prevention of most cancers.

The Role of Diet—Cancer Cells Lack Metabolic Flexibility

If cancer is caused by defective metabolism, then the first and most obvious treatment is through diet—after all, diet is the quickest and surest way to alter metabolism. It turns out that dramatically reducing the blood glucose that cancer cells so heavily rely upon both starves them and forces the body to generate new fuels from fat called ketones—a fuel source that cancer cells are unable to use because ketones can only be metabolized through oxidative pathways in the healthy fully-functional mitochondria of normal cells.

Normal cells of the body have metabolic flexibility. If glucose is unavailable, they can use either fatty acids or ketone bodies to provide energy. Cancer cells are unable to do this. They must have glucose. A Harvard research team found that depriving leukemia cancer cells of glucose caused them to die, whereas raising glucose levels resulted in favorable energy production in cancer cells.[14]

People who practice caloric restriction or periodic fasting have been shown to have lower cancer rates. Why? When calories are reduced to a certain threshold the body initiates a process called *autophagy* (self-digestion). Autophagy is a cellular process that acts as a repair mechanism by consuming damaged cellular components and uses the digested components to meet energy requirements. It also suppresses neoplasia by limiting inflammation and removing damaged mitochondria. The failure of autophagy is thought to be one of the main reasons for the accumulation of cell damage and aging.

But even though the dietary intake of glucose is low, the body will still make glucose via gluconeogenesis, and cancer cells are particularly efficient at stealing the little glucose available from the blood. So unless extreme, a carbohydrate restricted diet won't starve the cancer cells. Protein and fat can maintain the desired weight or be increased to gain weight when carbohydrates are restricted and muscles are exercised.

The Ketogenic Diet

A low-carbohydrate, ketogenic diet causes your body to enter ketosis. This means that your body is using fat for energy and blood levels of ketones are elevated. Ketones are burned for energy just like glucose. During the initial stage of ketosis, your blood glucose levels are maintained through gluconeogenesis. After about 48 hours, your body starts burning ketones from fat and reserving the limited amount of glucose available only for your absolute energy needs.

Low-carbohydrate ketogenic diets lead to low blood glucose levels and lower blood levels of the hormones insulin and IGF-1. The latter also may cause cancer cells to get less signals to divide and multiply. What's more, ketone bodies in themselves have been shown to inhibit the growth of cancer cells in laboratory cultures.[15] These findings about glucose deprivation and ketone toxicity have led to using ketogenic diets to inhibit and stop neoplasia.

In a 2011 pilot trial of 16 advanced-stage cancer patients, a ketogenic diet improved the quality of life and slowed the progression of cancer for the 5 patients who completed the 12-week study.[16]

A 2012 pilot study of 10 advanced cancer patients reported the results of a ketogenic diet for 28 days.[17] According to a PET scan, 4 of the patients continued to have progressive disease, while 5 remained stable and 1 had a partial remission. The patients who had the greatest positive metabolic response to the diet (that is, lowest insulin and highest ketone levels) saw the most improvement. That same year researchers at Barrow Neurological Institute at St. Joseph's Hospital and Medical Center reported effectively treating brain cancer patients using a combination of ketogenic diet and radiation therapy.

Researchers from the British Columbia Cancer Research Centre found that mice that ate a South Beach-like diet composed of 15 percent carbohydrates, 58 percent protein and 26 percent fat had slower tumor cell growth than mice that ate a typical Western diet of 55 percent carbohydrates, 23 percent protein and 22 percent fat.[18] Even though the study was in mice, researchers believed the findings were strong enough to have applications for humans.

Another study demonstrated that an insulin-inhibiting (ketogenic) diet is helpful in selected patients with advanced cancer.[19] The extent of ketosis, but not calorie deficit or weight loss, correlated with stable disease or partial remission. This suggests that adding ketones to a ketogenic diet might be beneficial.

Dr. Fred Hatfield is a case example of the efficacy of the ketogenic diet.[20] He is an impressive guy: a power-lifting champion, author of dozens of books and a millionaire businessman. But he'll tell you his greatest accomplishment is killing his cancer in the nick of time. "The doctors gave me three months to live because of widespread metastatic cancer in my skeletal structure," he recalled. "Three months—three different doctors told me that same thing." While Hatfield was preparing to die, he heard about an anti-cancer diet, also known as metabolic therapy. With nothing to lose, he gave it a try and was shocked when it actually worked. "The cancer was gone!" he exclaimed. "Completely. To this day there's no trace of it. And it's been over five years."

Although it wasn't easy, Hatfield was on a ketogenic diet. "Cancer cells love glucose and need it so badly, that if you stop giving it to them, they die. It just absolutely amazes me that medical science is just now finding this out," he said.

Hatfield's cancer recovery, however, was not a surprise to Dr. Dominic D'Agostino, who researches metabolic therapy. When he and his team of scientists at the University of South Florida removed carbohydrates from the diets of lab mice, the mice survived highly aggressive metastatic cancer longer than mice on a normal diet. The results were better than similar studies where mice were treated with chemotherapy. It's not just lab mice. Dr. D'Agostino also has seen similar success in humans. "I've been in correspondence with a number of people," he said. "At least a dozen over the last year-and-a-half to two years, and all of them are still alive, despite the odds. So this is very encouraging."[21]

"All cells, including cancer cells, are fueled by glucose. But if you deprive them of glucose, they switch to the alternate fuel, ketone bodies...except for cancer cells. A defect in cancer cells prevents them from making the switch to using ketone bodies as fuel and, therefore, they can only survive on glucose. All other cells can use either glucose or ketone bodies. Your normal cells have the metabolic flexibility to adapt from using glucose to using ketone bodies. But cancer cells lack this metabolic flexibility. So we can exploit that," Dr. D'Agostino explained.

Sometimes people are afraid to try the ketogenic diet because they think eating fat is bad for your heart. But more doctors say as long as it's natural, fat is good for you, even saturated fat like coconut oil and butter. "Is cholesterol the major cause of heart disease?" cardiologist Dr. Stephen Sinatra asked and answered, "Absolutely not." In his book *The Great Cholesterol Myth*,[22] Dr. Sinatra said the real cause of heart disease is inflammation, which comes from eating too many carbohydrates. "We need to coach our patients and empower our patients about the dangers of sugar," he said. "Unfortunately, they're not hearing that. They're hearing the converse, the dangers of fat. Fat is healthy for you, as long as you avoid trans fats. So by cutting back on carbohydrates and eating natural fats and proteins, you can improve your heart health and even wipe out cancer."

Sinatra pointed out that natural proteins are ones that are in their original form. In contrast, processed meats—like cold cuts and hot dogs—are off-limits because carbohydrates often have been added to them. Similarly, "natural" fats are whole foods, like olive oil, avocados and nuts. Stay away from "trans" fats, such as shortening or margarine and any oil that is hydrogenated. Trans fats are manufactured.

Dr. Sinatra's findings and recommendations were confirmed by Dr. Eric Westman and Jimmy Moore in their 2013 book *Cholesterol Clarity*.[23]

Adapting to this new metabolic state can be challenging for some people. The administration of ketone esters could conceivably enable them to reduce the dietary restriction generally required for sustained ketosis.[24] Ketone ester-induced ketosis would make sustained hypoglycemia more tolerable and thus assist in the metabolic management of cancer.

Artificial sweeteners may be associated with a variety of health problems from weight gain to headaches to mood changes to possibly cancer.[25] Stevia rebaudiana (stevia) is an acceptable and popular natural sweetener in the U.S. health food industry.

Nutrient Loaded Foods

Joel Fuhrman, M.D., author of *Eat for Health*, created rankings of foods according to the nutrients they pack—vitamins, minerals, antioxidants, etc., as measured by their Aggregate Nutrient Density Index (ANDI) scores assigned to foods that contain the highest nutrients per calorie.[26]

Nutritional science in the last twenty years has demonstrated that cruciferous plant foods, such as brussel sprouts, broccoli, cauliflower, Chinese cabbage and kale contain a huge assortment of protective compounds, most of which still remain unnamed. A study that tracked breast cancer for six years showed that those who consumed the most foods rich in carotenoids, such as carrots, sweet potatoes, tomatoes, apricots and beets lived longer than those who consumed less.[27] Tomatoes also contain other anticancer nutrients as shown in a study of prostate cancer, and kale appears to be especially effective in cancer prevention.[28] Only by eating an assortment of nutrient-rich natural foods can we access these protective compounds and prevent the common diseases that afflict us. Our modern, low-nutrient eating style has led to an overweight population, the majority of whom develop metabolic diseases. This is one of the reasons our health care costs are spiraling out of control.

Sample Nutrient/Calorie Density Scores					
Kale	1000	Cantalope	100	Skim Milk	36
Collards	1000	Kidney Beans	100	Walnuts	35
Bok Choy	824	Sweet Potato	83	Grapes	35
Spinach	739	Black Beans	83	White Potato	35
Brussel Sprouts	672	Apple	76	Banana	34
Swiss Chard	670	Peach	73	Whole Wheat Bread	30
Arugula	550	Green Peas	70	Low Fat Yogurt	28
Cabbage	481	Cherries	68	Cashews	27
Romaine Lettuce	389	Flax Seeds	65	Chicken Breast	24
Broccoli	376	Pineapple	64	Eggs	24
Carrot Juice	344	Chick Peas	57	Peanut butter	24
Cauliflower	295	Oatmeal	53	Feta Cheese	24
Green Peppers	258	Mango	51	Whole Milk	24
Artichoke	244	Cucumber	50	Ground Beef	21
Carrots	240	Soy Beans	48	White Pasta	16
Asparagus	234	Pistachio Nuts	48	White Bread	17
Strawberries	212	Corn	44	Apple Juice	14
Pomgranate Juice	193	Brown Rice	41	Swiss Cheese	14
Tomato	164	Salmon	39	Potato Chips	14
Blueberries	130	Almonds	38	American Cheese	14
Iceburg Lettuce	110	Shrimp	38	Vanilla Ice Cream	9
Orange	109	Avocado	37	French Fries	7
Lentils	100	Tofu	37	Cola	1
Adapted from: Dr. Fuhrman's Nutritarian Handbook & ANDI Food Scoring Guide					

Dr. Nyjon Eccles of The Chiron Clinic in London notes that plant-based phyto-nutrients decrease DNA damage, improve cell communication, improve cell detoxification, are anti-inflammatory, boost Immunity and improve circulation.[29] There may be other as yet undefined actions of phyto-nutrients that are relevant to their inhibitory effect on cancer.

Adding evidence for the nutritional approach, University of Southampton researchers have discovered a novel way of killing cancer cells that leaves healthy cells undamaged unlike conventional therapies.[30] Chris Proud, Professor of Cellular Regulation in Biological Sciences, said: "Cancer cells grow and divide much more rapidly than normal cells, meaning they have a much higher demand for and are often starved of nutrients." They discovered that a cellular component, eEF2K, plays a critical role in allowing cancer cells to survive nutrient starvation, while normal, healthy cells usually do not require eEF2K in order to survive. Therefore, by blocking the function of eEF2K, it may be possible to kill cancer cells without harming normal cells in the process. These researchers, in collaboration with colleagues at the British Columbia Cancer Agency Research Center, are now working with other laboratories, including pharmaceutical companies, to develop and test drugs that block eEF2K and could potentially be used to treat cancer.[31]

Carbonyl Compounds

Dr. William Koch's research in the 1950s focused on ways to return the body's oxidation mechanism back to its original vitality, thereby restoring the body's innate ability to maintain health in cancer and a host of other diseases.[32]

Dr. Koch's theories emphasized the relationship between environmental toxins, nutritional deficiencies and a depleted oxidation mechanism (the "Warburg effect") as primary initiators of the disease process. By studying the normal tissues that survived the longest in cancer patients, he found that the common feature was the presence of carbonyl compounds. He postulated that the toxic amines of various metabolic, bacterial, viral or fungal agents can cripple these important carbonyls and compromise the metabolic functions of cells.

Despite a number of cases of advanced cancers Koch treated successfully in the United States by the injection of Glyoxylide/Malonide that induced oxidation and a high fever intended to eradicate cancer through activation of one's own immune system, Dr. Koch was subjected to criticism from organized medicine and inconclusive legal action by the Food and Drug Administration from 1923 to 1943, leading him to leave the United States in 1948.[33]

In 1963, Dr. Szent-Gyorgyi also wrote about the anti-neoplastic action of carbonyl compounds and how they can arrest cell division.[34] His research suggested that these substances are not only able to inhibit cell proliferation but also to maintain cells in a normal oxidative metabolism. He suggested that the body can lose or become compromised in its ability to produce these substances thereby encouraging the development of cancer. Further research on carbonyl and cancer has not been noticeably reported.

Anti-angiogenic Foods

Anti-angiogenic therapies stop the growth of tumors and progression of cancers by limiting the formation of new blood vessels in cancer tumors (angiogenesis). They have been a factor in the improved survival of people with kidney cancer, multiple myeloma, colorectal cancer and gastrointestinal stromal tumors. That's impressive. But for other cancer types, the improvements have only been modest.

So Dr. William Li of the Angiogenesis Foundation asked, "Why haven't we been able to do better?"[35] Could the answer to cancer be preventing angiogenesis so the cancers could never become dangerous? This could help healthy people as well as people who've already beaten cancer and want to find a way to keep it from coming back. To look for a way to prevent angiogenesis in cancer, Li went back to look at cancer's causes. What intrigued him was his finding that diet accounts for one-third of environmentally caused cancers.

What could we add to our diet that's naturally anti-angiogenic and that could boost the body's defense system and beat back those blood vessels that are feeding cancer tumors? In other words, can we eat to starve cancer blood vessels? Resveratrol found in red wine inhibits abnormal angiogenesis by 60 percent. A growing list of anti-angiogenic foods and beverages includes strawberries, soybeans, parsley, garlic, tomatoes and four different teas: Chinese jasmine, Japanese sencha, Earl Grey and a blend that is more potent than either one alone. This suggests that combining anti-angiogenic foods might have merit.

What is the evidence that eating certain foods can reduce angiogenesis in cancer? Well, the best example is a study of 79,000 men followed over 20 years, in which it was found that men who consumed cooked tomatoes two to three times a week had up to a 50 percent reduction in their risk of developing prostate cancer.[36] We know that tomatoes are a good source of lycopene, and lycopene is anti-angiogenic. But what's even more interesting from this study is that in those men who did develop prostate cancer, those who ate more servings of tomato sauce actually had fewer blood vessels feeding their cancer. So this human study is a prime example of how anti-angiogenic substances present in food and consumed at practical levels can have impact on cancer.

Coenzyme Q10 (CoQ10)/Ubiquinol

Coenzyme Q10 was discovered by Professor Fredrick L. Crane and colleagues at the University of Wisconsin–Madison Enzyme Institute in 1957. The highest concentration of CoQ10 is found on the inner membrane of the mitochondria of your cells.

In the 1980s, numerous scientists around the globe started studying CoQ10 in relation to various diseases, including cardiovascular diseases and cancer. Interest in it as a potential therapeutic agent in cancer was stimulated by an observational study that found that individuals with lung, pancreas and especially breast cancer were more likely to have low plasma CoQ10 levels than healthy controls. Although the benefit of CoQ10 is best documented in the treatment of heart failure, two studies suggest promise in the treatment of cancer.

In 1994, Knud Lockwood, a cancer specialist in Copenhagen, described his treatment of 32 "high-risk" breast cancer patients with antioxidant vitamins, essential fatty acids and CoQ10 (200-400 mg. daily).[37] "No patient died and all expressed a feeling of well-being," he wrote "These clinical results are remarkable...After 24 months, all still survived; about 6 deaths would have been expected." Six of the 32 patients showed partial tumor remission, and two benefited from very high doses of CoQ10. One, a 59-year-old woman with a family history of breast cancer, had a tumor recurrence, but one month after increasing her CoQ10 intake to 400 mg. daily the tumor disappeared. Another patient, age 74, had a small tumor removed from her right breast. She refused a second operation to remove additional growths and began taking 300 mg. of CoQ10 daily. Three months later, mammography revealed no evidence of the tumor or metastases. Lockwood, who apparently treated some 7,000 cases of breast cancer over 35 years, wrote that until using CoQ10, he had "never seen a spontaneous complete regression of a 1.5-2.0 centimeter breast tumor, and had never seen a comparable regression on any conventional anti-tumor therapy."

In 1997, Dr. Karl Folkers of the University of Texas-Austin described ten cancer patients given CoQ10 for heart failure. One of the patients, a 48-year-old man diagnosed with inoperable lung cancer, had no signs of either cancer or heart failure symptoms while taking CoQ10 for 17 years.[38] In 1999, Dr. Hodges reported an uncontrolled trial suggesting that coenzyme Q10 supplementation may be beneficial as an adjunct to conventional therapy for breast cancer.[39]

Antioxidants (a misleading term because they do not remove oxygen) are molecules that can safely remove free radicals before they damage cells. Free radicals, also called reactive oxygen species (ROS), are atoms or groups of atoms with an odd (unpaired) number of electrons that can be formed when oxygen interacts with certain molecules. Oxygen itself can become a ROS when it loses electrons and becomes a "superoxide anion". ROS are formed naturally in the body. In addition, environmental toxins in polluted air and food additives may stimulate the body's cells to produce more ROS that are highly reactive and have the potential to cause damage to cells, including damage that may lead to cancer.[40] CoQ10's role as your body's natural, powerful antioxidant and immune system stimulant that removes ROS probably is responsible for its benefits in aging, cancer and other diseases. Its antioxidant effect comes from the CoQ10 molecule quite easily giving up electrons and, thus, restoring electrons in ROS. It is more effective than other antioxidants, especially in its active form in the body: ubiquinol.

Fluctuating levels of blood glucose as seen in obesity and diabetes can produce ROS.[41] Once formed these highly reactive radicals can start a chain domino-like reaction. The chief danger comes from the damage they can do when they react with important cellular components, such as

DNA or the cell membrane. Cells may die or function poorly and enter neoplasia when this occurs.

Antioxidants can inhibit the development of cancer cells caused by ROS, but cancer cells themselves are susceptible to die from high levels of ROS. One strategy in chemotherapy is to increase the oxidative stress of cancer cells by exposing them to ROS. Antioxidants might well interfere with this form of chemotherapy. They also might reduce the general oxidative stress on cancer cells and encourage their growth.[42] It turns out that at a certain level of ROS can help the immune system kill infections and cancer cells, so both too many and too few ROS spell trouble.[43] Many oncologists recommend avoiding CoQ10 and other antioxidant supplements during chemotherapy and radiation therapy. At the same time CoQ10—preferably taken in its active form in the body as ubiquinol—has been reported to reduce the side effects of chemotherapies that do not increase the oxidative stress on cancer cells.[44]

The principle antioxidant nutrients in foods are vitamin E, beta-carotene and vitamin C. Selenium, a trace metal that is required for proper function of one of the body's antioxidant enzyme systems, is sometimes included in this category. Green tea also contains an antioxidant. Trials of beta-carotene with lung and vitamin E and selenium with prostate cancer patients were stopped because they appeared to increase the progress of cancer.[45] It is possible that the lack of benefit in clinical studies of tested antioxidants, such as beta-carotene, vitamin E, alpha-tocopherol, and selenium, can be explained by differences in the effects when they are consumed as purified chemicals as opposed to when they are consumed in foods, which contain complex mixtures of other antioxidants, vitamins and minerals.[46] In contrast to these chemicals, CoQ10 in the form of ubiquinol is a naturally occurring antioxidant in your body.

Putting all of this information together leads to the conclusion that ubiquinol can play an important role in preventing cancer by keeping ROS levels in your body in balance. Because CoQ10 levels decrease with aging, ubiquinol also has demonstrated anti-aging properties.[47] Whether or not it is contraindicated in persons with cancer, especially

while receiving chemotherapy, is controversial and warrants individualized judgments.

Vitamin B17

Dr. Jay F. Hoffman, the author of the book *Hunza—Secrets Of The
World's Healthiest And Oldest Living People* published in 1960 was sent to
Hunza under the auspices of the American Geriatrics Society.[48] Hunza
then was an area slightly more than a hundred miles long and wide in the
Himalayan Mountains of Pakistan with approximately thirty thousand
inhabitants.

The Hunzas apparently have been cancer free for over 900 years of
their existence. They have a natural diet and are comparatively free of
toxic chemicals in the air and water. Coming from glaciers, their water
has an alkaline pH, deuterium depletion, negative Redox potential and
a high colloidal mineral content. Their diet does not include white rice,
white flour, sugar and, for the most part, meat. Instead, they eat locally
grown organic fruit, vegetables, unprocessed fresh milk products and
green or whole grains. They engage in regular meditative practices and
exercise.

The Hunzas eat fresh apricots for the three months they are in sea-
son, and the remainder of the year they eat dried apricots, including their
seeds. This supplies them with 50 to 75 milligrams of Vitamin B17 a day.

The Hunza people live to be 100, 110, 120 and not uncommonly 140
years of age. Here is a land where people have not been plagued by the
diseases of the Western world.[49] Moreover, when they began to be studied
in the 1950s there were no hospitals, no mental hospitals, no drug stores,
no saloons, no tobacco stores, no police, no jails, no crimes, no murders
and no beggars.

In spite of its suggestive value in treating cancer, Vitamin B17 is
controversial because clinical studies have not upheld its value, and toxic
effects from its breakdown into cyanide that may take place when ingested
have been reported.[50]

When it is used for cancer, most experts recommend a daily dose of apricot kernels from between 24 up to 40 kernels spread throughout a day. For a person in remission, 16 apricot kernels a day would be a minimum.

Acidity vs Alkalinity

Testing the pH of your saliva is desirable in general and especially if you have cancer. Litmus strips can be purchased at any drug store.

The pH of your tissues and body fluids mirrors the state of your health and your inner "cleanliness." The closer the pH is to 7.35-7.45, the higher your level of health and wellbeing. The most important reason for this is that all of the proteins that work in your body need to maintain a specific geometric shape to function. Their three-dimensional shapes are affected by tiny changes in the pH of your body fluids. Staying within this range presumably increases your ability to resist acute illnesses like a cold and the flu as well as the onset of cancer and other diseases.

Deviations above or below a 7.35-7.45 pH range can signal potentially serious body states. When your body can no longer effectively neutralize and eliminate acids, it relocates them within your body's extra-cellular fluids and connective tissue cells and directly compromises cellular integrity. Conversely, when your body becomes too alkaline, metabolic alkalosis occurs, which can lead to severe consequences if not corrected quickly. Keeping your body pH within a healthy range is a good idea over the long term.

Cancer grows in an acidic environment (low pH), and acidity helps neoplasia and enables cancer cells to spread. Dr. Mark Pagel at the University of Arizona Cancer Center is testing the effects of sodium bicarbonate in treating neoplasia by measuring the pH of a tumor with a MRI machine and then testing the effect of sodium bicarbonate on the cancer cells.[51] He found it selectively increased the pH of tumors and reduced the formation of spontaneous metastases in mouse models of metastatic breast cancer. Sodium bicarbonate is a possible treatment option, but only if a tumor is determined to be acidic by using a special MRI.

The vast majority of highly processed foods—like white flour products and white sugar—have an acidic effect on your body and will overwork your body's pH buffering systems. If you're eating mainly grains, flour products and meat and washing these foods down with coffee, soda and milk, you will almost certainly improve your health by replacing some of your food and beverage choices with fresh vegetables and other nutrient-dense foods. Paradoxically, fresh lemon juice is acidic until it enters the body where it is alkalizing. If you are on a restricted ketogenic diet and your pH goes down, Red Desert Clay can alkalinize your body and remove toxins and minerals as well.

Traditional Chinese Medicine

Ideas about health and illness developed much differently in Asia than in the Western world. In Asia illness is seen as an imbalance in complicated forces within the body that produces symptoms. Accordingly, treatments usually involve concoctions of ingredients that have different effects in the body and work synergistically to produce a greater effect than any single ingredient could do. For example, acupuncture is based on the concept that the body has multiple points along its energy channels for targeting treatment.

According to the American Cancer Society, There is evidence from randomized clinical trials that some Chinese herbs may contribute to longer survival rates, reduction of side effects and lower risk of recurrence for some types of cancer, especially when combined with conventional treatment.

A large scale review of research on Traditional Chinese Medicine (TCM) by Australia's University of Western Sydney and the Beijing University of Chinese Medicine disclosed that it offers significant benefits for most types of cancers.[52] Researchers reviewed 2,964 human clinical studies and found that 72% of them applied TCM alongside conventional treatment. In 1,015 studies TCM treatment resulted in improvement of cancer symptoms with many reporting reduced pain. In another 883 studies, 70% showed increased survival rates.

Soy is regarded as an anticancer nutrient. A study reported that

Chinese women who consumed more soy before being diagnosed with lung cancer lived longer compared with those who consumed less soy.[53]

Artemisinin, a chemical isolated from sweet wormwood, has potent anti-malarial activity. It is being developed as an anti-cancer therapeutic agent as well. The advantage of artemisinin as an anti-cancer agent is not only its potency as a toxic agent to cancer cells, but also its selectivity in killing cancer cells and low toxicity to normal cells.[54]

Oxygen Therapy

The evidence is clear that cancer cells don't need oxygen. Based on reviews of the literature, there's evidence that hyperbaric oxygen might have tumor-inhibitory effects in certain cancer subtypes.[55] There's no evidence that hyperbaric oxygen stimulates tumor growth nor enhances cancer recurrence.

CELLFOOD is a line of health supplements developed and marketed by NuScience Corp. NuScience says that CELLFOOD increases oxygen at the cellular level and enhances your body's metabolic functions. Additionally, NuScience claims that Cellfood can detoxify your body and increase your energy by transporting oxygen to your cells. It also has anti-oxidant and alkalinizing properties. For over forty-five years, CELLFOOD (Deutrosulfazyme) has safely provided nutritional benefits and more recently has been shown to suppress and kill cancer cells.[56] Cancer cells thrive in an acidic body and can't stand high levels of oxygen.

Genetic vs Lifestyle Factors

There's a lot of talk about genes and family history in cancer, as though it's predetermined from the day you are born whether or not you will get cancer. Aside from instilling unnecessary fear in many people, this mode of thinking leaves you powerless to do anything but sit and wait to get sick and actually is inaccurate.

In reality, your genes typically have little to do with your likelihood of getting any disease with some rare exceptions. Your genes are merely storage facilities, and they have no intelligence whatsoever. What is important, however, is the expression of your genes by the stimuli that actually cause your DNA to replicate proteins. Your physical environment, diet, life experiences, thoughts and emotions (and let's not forget your stress levels) and life style choices influence the expression of your genes through what is called epigenesis.

This point was supported by Dean Ornish's studies of men with early low grade prostate cancer who declined surgery, hormonal therapy and radiation and instead participated in an intensive nutrition and life style intervention while undergoing careful surveillance for tumor progression.[57] These men made changes in their diets, exercised moderately, used stress management techniques and participated in a support group. The program consisted of a vegetarian, non-dairy diet supplemented with antioxidants (such as lycopene, selenium and vitamin E), moderate aerobic exercise and stress management techniques. This diet suppressed blood glucose levels and tumor progression. Prostate cancer cell growth was inhibited almost eight times as much in the experimental group compared to the control group. At a five-year follow-up it was associated with telomere lengthening rather than expected normal telomere shortening from aging in the chromosomes of immune system cells. This suggests an anti-aging effect of the diet as well.

The Inuit Indians in Canada ate a diet high in meat and fat, low in fruits and vegetables and still had low rates of heart disease and cancer. When more modernization came to them in the form of convenience stores, soda and other processed foods these diseases started to increase.[58]

Cancer Prevention

The scientific evidence reveals that neoplasia is a chronic, metabolic disease linked with our diets and environmental exposures. Most metabolic diseases have specific vitamins and minerals as their basis. The most familiar is scurvy—a fatal disease that wiped out an entire Polar expedition and accounted for high mortality among the Crusaders. Prior to the incorporation of Vitamin C into their diets, it wasn't uncommon for three-fourths of a ship's crew to become seriously ill by the end of a long voyage and then those who didn't die would mysteriously recover after hitting shore because they would have access to fresh fruits and vegetables rich in Vitamin C.

Pernicious anemia had a mortality rate of 98 percent until a very simple remedy for preventing and curing this disease was discovered... raw liver, which contains vitamin B12 and folic acid. Another metabolic disease is pellagra that is completely prevented and cured by Brewer's yeast containing niacin—vitamin B3.

The biological experience of the human organism over the millions of years of evolution consisted of exposure to water, air, carbohydrates, fats, amino acids and various salts that became parts of the evolving organism. We need to look at our devitalized food and attempt to replace that which was removed from it in the process of food refining, manipulation or cooking.

Viewing cancer as a multitude of separate diseases makes its prevention seem hopeless. On the other hand, recognizing that cancer cells are the result of neoplasia—a dysfunction in the metabolism and life cycle of cells offers a hopeful model for prevention.

Although it seems far-fetched now, it's not out of the realm of possibility that cancer could be prevented through nutritional means, just as we prevent scurvy, pernicious anemia and pellagra. At the very least, we do know that nutrition plays a role in the prevention and treatment of cancer. Already we know that cruciferous vegetables and Omega 3 containing foods reduce inflammation and the risk of several forms of cancer.[59] Chapter Fifteen provides details about cancer causing agents that can be avoided. It is not out of the realm of possibility that nutrition could even counteract the effects of environmental toxins.

Conclusion

Given that glucose reducing diets can drastically improve and even cure some diseases, it doesn't take a stretch of the imagination to see how these diets may reduce chances of developing cancer later in life. The elevated blood sugar and insulin levels seen in diabetes and the inflammation that accompanies obesity already are known risk factors for cancer that can be reduced on a low carbohydrate diet.

Strikingly, nutritional therapy for cancer has not been subjected to rigorous...and costly...clinical studies in the way that chemotherapies have. It is evident that there are few, if any, financial incentives to study nutritional therapy that can be carried out by patients themselves with minimal professional participation and without expenditures for drugs, equipment and facilities. This is unfortunate since patients have been deprived of studies assessing the effectiveness, or lack of effectiveness, of dietary changes that could help them combat their cancer. Fortunately, clinical trials of the ketogenic diet in cancer are beginning to be conducted.

We are left with the need to personally explore nutritional therapies and judge for ourselves whether or not they are worth trying. If traditional radiation and chemotherapy effectively cured cancer or even substantially extended high qualities of life, the nutritional approach would be less appealing. Even then, if the same, or better, results can be obtained through nutritional adjustments, the preponderance of the evidence suggests that they are worth trying to complement conventional therapies.

Even in the context of conventional cancer treatment the sequence of 1) surgery or radiation for removing or ablating identifiable malignancies, 2) nutritional therapy, and then 3) chemotherapy and/or radiation, if needed, makes clinical and ethical sense. The fact that traditional chemotherapy and radiation have harmful side-effects—some devastating—creates an incentive to try nutritional therapy before employing them in the early stages of cancer. The most promising nutritional therapies for cancer are the ketogenic diet that may starve cancer cells, increasing intracellular oxygen and curcumin that has multiple anti-cancer properties as outlined in the following chapter.

Chapter Eleven

What You Can Do Now to Complement Your Cancer Treatment

Key complementary therapies for cancer are described.

Throughout history, natural products have found many applications in medicine, pharmacology and biology. A number of important commercialized drugs have been obtained from natural sources or by designing new compounds with natural compounds as models. In treating cancer, natural products can be more effective and cost much less than modern anti-cancer drugs.[1] How to take advantage of them is the perplexing question.

As you explore ways to enhance your cancer treatment, you will encounter bewildering claims of secret and well-known ingredients that presumably will cure your cancer. You will find non-mainstream cancer clinics and hospitals that claim remarkable results, if not cures, for cancer supported by testimonials from patients who have benefited from their approaches for decades. You, as do I, will wonder why, if they have had such outstanding results, they have not collected data and published reports so that mainstream medicine could evaluate their claims and everyone could benefit from their approaches. The bottom line is that desperate people with cancer are especially vulnerable to exploitation and to outright quackery. For this reason, it is important to exercise caution and evaluate the treatment options available to you.

First of all, "alternative", "complementary" and "integrative" medicine are terms you will encounter as you seek to take charge of your cancer care. "Alternative" medicine refers to a non-mainstream approach to health maintenance or health problems. "Complementary" medicine refers to using a non-mainstream approach together with conventional medicine. "Integrative" mainstream health care providers integrate alternative practices into conventional treatments and promoting health. For example, guided imagery, acupuncture, yoga and massage once considered "complementary" or "alternative" are used in "integrative" cancer centers to help patients manage pain and other discomforts. Some alternative treatments are used for symptom control rather than direct cancer treatment. As examples, yoga, reiki and acupuncture may help improve a cancer patient's quality of life, while therapies like lymphatic massage and hyperbaric oxygen may reduce the side effects of cancer treatment.

The National Center for Complementary and Alternative Medicine (NCCAM) is the Federal Government's lead agency for scientific research on health interventions, practices, products and disciplines that originate from outside mainstream medicine. The NCCAM says that nearly forty percent of Americans use health care approaches developed outside of conventional medicine for specific conditions or for overall well-being.

A misconception about alternative treatments is that if they really worked doctors everywhere would be using them. Actually and understandably, doctors rely upon tried and true treatments and new therapies that have been proved to work. Unfortunately, the kind of scientific evidence that is sufficient to lead to FDA approval is extremely expensive to produce. This means that only entities that can afford to spend millions of dollars on research can undertake basic research and clinical studies. There is no financial incentive to test nutritional or non-patentable agents.

The separation of alternative (naturopathic) and conventional (allopathic) medicine has stood in the way of drawing upon and combining the best in both fields. This means you need to do your own homework in order to make decisions about your treatment. However, a lack of reliable data makes it difficult for anyone to make informed decisions.

What's more, it is likely that life style is a contributing factor in the development of cancer. For this reason, persons with cancer need to change their life styles if they wish to shift their outlooks from the chances of a five-year survival with conventional treatment to a life without cancer. This means adopting a life style with health inducing nutrition, exercise and stress reducing practices. It really boils down to how much personal responsibility and attendant inconvenience and sacrifice you are willing to accept in order to have a life free of neoplasia produced cancer cells.

Although written for everyone as a way to prevent cancer, Dr. David Servan-Schreiber's book *Anticancer: A New Way of Life* is an excellent background for adopting a life style that can favorably complement your cancer treatment. The book outlines basic principles for a healthy diet, reducing exposure to carcinogenic toxins and maintaining an optimal mind-body balance.[2] It also offers advice about avoiding charlatans. They should be suspected when they:

+ Offer secret formulas that entail purchasing their literature and products;
+ Recommend stopping conventional treatments;
+ Do not work in collaboration with other professionals;
+ Do not have evidence to support their claims other than testimonials;
+ Suggest a treatment whose price is out of proportion to likely benefits; and
+ Promise that their approach will work if you have a true desire to recover.

Complementary Treatments

In order to try to help you evaluate alternative treatments for cancer, I intensively explored non-mainstream approaches and selected from the array of alternative therapies the following as the most scientifically

> ### Complementary Cancer Treatment Protocol
>
> Ketogenic diet
> CELLFOOD
> Curcumin
> Immpower (AHCC)
> Milk thistle (silymarin)
> Aspirin
> Vitamin D3
> Stress relieving meditation
> Exercise
> Support system—media and/or interpersonal

justified and efficacious and categorized them according to their mode of action. If you are seeking treatment for advanced cancer, the most effective approach is to use all of them as a "cocktail" because of the possible synergetic effects they might have, as suggested by Dr. Raymond Chang in his book *Beyond the Magic Bullet: The Anti-cancer Cocktail*.[3] Dr. Chang offers suggestions for a wide variety of additional alternative agents.

Although all of the following agents are generally safe and without significant side effects, it is advisable to check with your doctor before using any of them to be sure that they do not conflict with the management of your specific medical conditions. To obtain maximum benefit, they all should be drawn upon as a multi-system "anti-cancer cocktail".

1) Destroy existing cancer cells

a) *Cancer cells require glucose and will starve without it.* There is substantial evidence that a *ketogenic diet* will starve existing cancer cells.[4] Normal cells can live well on ketone bodies that are produced when you are on a low carbohydrate diet; cancer cells cannot. Several studies also have shown that a ketogenic diet is well-tolerated and reduces chemotherapy and radiation-induced side effects in patients with advanced cancer.[5]

Here are examples of ketogenic diets that will reduce carbohydrate intake so that your body will go into ketosis and shift from glucose to ketone bodies for energy:

- ◆ Kalamian, Miriam (2014) Get Started with the Ketogenic Diet for Cancer. Hamilton, MT: Dietary Therapies.
- ◆ Ellen Davis (2013) *Fight Cancer with a Ketogenic Diet.* www. ketogenic-diet-resource.com.
- ◆ Eric Westman (2013) *A Low Carbohydrate, Ketogenic Diet Manual: No Sugar, No Starch Diet.* www.amazon.com.
- ◆ Dana Carpender (2002) *500 Low-Carb Recipes: 500 Recipes from Snacks to Dessert, That the Whole Family Will Love.* http:// holdthetoast.com/low_carb_books_by_dana_carpender.

Because there is evidence that ketone bodies in themselves adversely affect cancer cells, adding a 600 mg capsule of the coconut oil ketone producing derivative *caprylic acid* twice daily to a ketogenic diet may be beneficial. Another consideration is that cow's milk may promote inflammation (and thus neoplasia).[6] Soy milk that includes calcium supplementation is an alternative to cow's milk. Almond milk provides calcium in amounts equivalent to cow's milk.

You can determine when you enter ketosis (this is not the same as diabetic ketosis and takes place usually in about three days) by a simple urine strip test available over the counter in drug stores. It helps you to know that you are in ketosis and to maintain the diet. This method of ketone testing is not as accurate as a blood test but can be used to determine if you have entered ketosis. After several weeks on the diet, your body converts most of the ketones for which the urine strips test (acetoacetate) to another type of ketone (beta-hydroxybutyrate), so that urine strips won't detect ketones as accurately after that. This means that a high level of ketones in urine testing may drop to a lower level without actually reflecting a decrease in circulating ketones.

A ketone screening kit contains plastic film like matchsticks with a pad.

i)   Remove one of the sticks and immediately close the lid of the container because even a very small amount of moisture can affect how the testing works.

ii) Totally immerse the pad at the end of the strip in urine collected in a clean, dry glass or in the urinating stream. Immediately remove it so the pad does not dissolve.

iii) Hold the testing strip horizontally and wait for exactly 15 seconds. When the color on the testing strip changes, check the color against the color chart provided in the kit. The color chart will tell you whether you have ketones in your urine, as well as an approximate level. A desirable level is 40-80 mg/dl (moderate to low large range).

If you are so inclined, following your blood sugar and ketone levels can give you more precise information about your progress. In her book *Fight Cancer with a Ketogenic Diet: A New Method for Treating Cancer*, Ellen Davis describes how monitoring blood glucose and ketone body levels can be done with a glucose/ketone meter such as the Precision Xtra by Abbott Laboratories or the Nova Max Plus from Nova Diabetes Care. Many persons with diabetes routinely test their blood with an easy finger pin prick this way. The meters are inexpensive, but the strips are not. To save money, shopping for glucose and ketone strips on the internet is advisable. Assistance in learning how to take your blood sugar and ketone readings is posted on: http://www.ketogenic-diet-resource.com/checking-blood-sugar.html.

Blood glucose readings should be taken before breakfast, two hours after lunch and a final daily reading two hours after the evening meal once or twice a week. Daily readings for the first week or two will give you a useful baseline. Keeping a food log and recording blood sugar and ketone readings initially is recommended so the effect of food choices can be detected, tracked and adjusted to meet target values. The other benefit of logging food intake and blood readings is having this information available for health care professionals, especially if you are having trouble reaching blood glucose or ketone target levels.

Recently, metformin, widely prescribed for diabetes, has been sup-ported by epidemiological, preclinical and clinical evidence for use in the treatment of cancer to enhance a ketogenic diet because it reduces blood sugar levels.[7] It's being tested in clinical trials as both a treatment for can-cer and to prevent it in people at increased risk for cancer, including cancer survivors who have a higher risk of recurrence. The National Cancer Institute is collaborating with the National Institute of Diabetes and Digestive and Kidney Diseases in a landmark clinical trial, the Diabetes Prevention Program, to investigate metformin's impact on cancer.[8] You will need a prescription to add metformin to your ketogenic diet to reduce your blood glucose levels and simultaneously give you more flexibility in your diet.

A bonus of the ketogenic diet is removing the stress on your brain caused by wheat, carbohydrates and sugar as described in Dr. David Permutter's book *Grain Brain: The Surprising Truth about Wheat, Carbs, and Sugar-Your Brain's Silent Killers.*[9]

Adhering to a ketogenic diet is not easy, especially for those of us who "live to eat." This why motivation to "starve cancer cells" with the goal of shifting from a future of a chance for a five-year survival to a life without cancer is essential.

b) *Cancer cells thrive in an acidic body and can't stand high levels of oxygen.* (You should test your salivary pH first thing in the morning and/or 2 hours after meals with strips available in health food stores to see if it is acidic.) Regulating the pH balance of your body is the first line of defense for your immune system. Bacteria, viruses, fungi and cancer cells multiply faster in acidic blood and are deterred by a blood pH between 6.8 and 7.4.

Low oxygen levels have been shown to cause uncontrollable growth in some forms of cancer, and deuterium-depleted water is used in Hungary to increase the oxygen levels in cells in the treatment of cancer.[10] Healthy cells quickly adapt to increased oxygen, but cancer cells are unable to do so. It is essential to complement a ketogenic diet with an agent that both normalizes your body pH and increases oxygen in your body's cells as does CELLFOOD™.

For over forty-five years, CELLFOOD (Deutrosulfazyme) has safely provided nutritional benefits and more recently has been shown to suppress and kill cancer cells.[11] CELLFOOD provides oxygen and essential nutrients to your body at the cellular level by breaking down the water molecule into hydrogen and oxygen. It contains 17 amino acids, 34 enzymes, 78 minerals and trace elements, deuterons, electrolytes and dissolved oxygen. It cleanses your body of toxins and acidic wastes as well as creating energy. Because it expels a small percentage of energy in tap water, for maximum benefit it should be taken with purified water (distilled or reverse osmotic) or natural fruit juices.

CELLFOOD is available at health food stores and on the internet.[12]

If your early morning salivary pH remains acidic on this program, among the best ways to raise it to the desirable level of 6.8-7.4 is to drink water laced with cod liver oil and/or alkaline capsules, such as Pine's International alfalfa (available at health stores), or to imbibe the juice of lemons or limes (even though acidic, they actually increase body pH).

c) *Hyperbaric oxygen also is being used to ensure that adequate levels of oxygen get into the blood stream and cells.* The usual protocol is 90 minutes in an oxygen chamber a week for six weeks, two weeks off and then six weeks again. This routine is repeated as necessary. Professional guidance and prescription is necessary for this treatment.[13]

d) *Curcumin can inhibit tumor growth and metastasis.* The United States has almost 3 times as many cases of cancer as in India. The death rate of persons with cancer in India is 60% of that in the United States.[14] This has been attributed to the prevalence of curry in the Indian diet. Turmeric is the main component of most curry blends and the ingredient of mustard that gives it its yellow color. It contains curcumin that has been shown to selectively kill tumor cells and not normal cells in leukemia and lymphoma, gastrointestinal cancers, genitourinary cancers, breast cancer, ovarian cancer, head and neck squamous cell carcinoma, lung cancer, melanoma, neurological cancers and sarcomas.[15] Curcumin acts through seven anti-cancer pathways. It also may protect normal cells from the toxic effects of chemotherapy drugs and radiation.[16]

Curcumin is not easy for your body to absorb if it is not in highly spicy foods. For optimal benefit a proprietary complex CuraMed delivers 7 to 10 times more curcumin to the bloodstream than plain curcumin. Its usual dosage is one or two 750 mg. softgels a day with meals. Studies haven't shown any toxicity up to 10 grams of plain curcumin a day that even can be administered intravenously by physicians. Curcumin has blood thinning properties and should be used only with your doctor's supervision if you are taking an anticoagulant. It also may increase the effects of stomach acid reducing and diabetes medications.[17]

d) *Boost your immune system so that it can improve its cancer cell detecting and removing capacity.* The mushroom product immpower (AHCC) is an immune system modulator supported by 20 human clinical studies, by over 30 papers published in PubMed-indexed journals and by more than 100 pre-clinical and in vitro studies.[18] An extract from hybridized medicinal mushrooms grown in rice bran, AHCC has been shown to increase the production of Natural Killer T Cells. Currently used in over 700 clinics throughout Asia, the most important factor driving the acceptance of AHCC has been its impact on reducing the side effects of chemotherapy. For maximum benefit take two 500 mg. capsules per day with each meal.

f) *Draw upon the multiple effects of Milk thistle (silymarin).* Laboratory studies demonstrate that silymarin functions as an antioxidant, stimulates detoxification pathways, stimulates regeneration of liver tissue, inhibits the growth of and kills certain cancer cell lines, and may increase the efficacy and decrease the toxicity of chemotherapy agents.[19] Few adverse side effects have been reported. The standard dose is 250 mg. once or twice daily.

2)   Prevent the formation of cancer cells

a) *Inflammation is an established factor in causing neoplasia and the development of cancer cells.* A growing body of evidence suggests that aspirin at regular dosages may be useful in preventing the formation of cancer cells. Among women living at least 1 year after a breast cancer diagnosis, aspirin use was associated with a decreased risk of metastasis and breast cancer death.[20] However, for the same reason that aspirin helps prevent strokes and heart attacks—reducing the blood's tendency to clot—it also raises the risk of bleeding elsewhere in the body. Aspirin also blocks the effects of chemicals that protect the stomach and gastrointestinal tract from damage. Bufferin may minimize these symptoms. These factors should be considered for the long-term use of aspirin.

b) *Low levels of vitamin D have been linked to certain kinds of cancers as well as to diabetes and asthma.* Recent research suggests that vitamin D3 can prevent cancer and even kill human cancer cells as well.[21] Dosages of 4,000-8,000 IU daily are recommended for this purpose. Because multivitamin and calcium supplements, which are desirable in general, already contain Vitamin D3, their levels should be counted in your daily intake. Too much Vitamin D3 can raise calcium levels to an excessively high level. Your doctor can obtain your serum 1,25-dihyroxy D3 level to determine what dosage is appropriate for you.

c) *Remove toxic substances from your body.* There are a number of diets designed for this purpose. Terramin is a simple option made from calcium montmorillonite clay.[22] It's a powerful trace mineral supplement containing a combination of more than 60 essential trace mineral elements in their natural forms. It presumably removes pathogens, heavy metals and toxins ingested from food grown in our chemically saturated fields from your colon. It restores minerals lacking in our overburdened depleted soil and has been used for centuries by Native Americans to restore health in a variety of conditions.

One pattern for using Terramin is to take it for a week initially. Thereafter, taking it for three or four days monthly may suffice to remove toxins from your body.

Do not take Terramin with meals, other supplements or with prescription drugs. Because of its detoxification properties, it may compete with your body in absorbing the other things you are taking. Wait at least 2 hours after meals and taking other supplements. Many people prefer to take it at bedtime.

3)   Relieve Stress and a Sense of Helplessness

a) *Stress contributes to neoplasia and undermines chemotherapy.* Chapter Twelve outlines ways of dealing with stress. More specifically, in his book *The Healing Power of Sound,* Dr. Mitchell Gaynor, an integrative oncologist, shows how, when a part of a mind-body-spirit approach to wellness, music can play a significant part in healing cancer.[23] Numerous studies have demonstrated the health benefits of music. It can lower blood pressure and heart and respiratory rates; reduce cardiac complications; increase your immune response; and boost your natural opiates. Dr. Gaynor's book includes twelve exercises involving breathing, meditation and "toning"—using pure vocal sound to resolve tension, release emotion and spur the healing process—that can be used by anyone to improve health and quality of life. Quartz singing bowls are especially soothing and conducive to meditation.

At least 25-30% of persons with cancer and an even higher percentage of those in an advanced stage meet the criteria for a psychiatric diagnosis. Psychoactive medications can alleviate cancer-related symptoms, such as pain, itching, nausea and vomiting, fatigue, cognitive impairment and hot flashes.[24]

b) *Exercise can help prevent and treat cancer by strengthening your immune system.* The latest research shows that exercise for cancer patients may keep cancer from recurring.[25] Your exercise program should be based on what's safe and works best for you. The goal is to stay as active and fit as possible. If you exercised before treatment, you need to adapt your exercise to surgery, radiation or chemotherapy. People who were sedentary before cancer treatment may need to start with short, low-intensity activity, such as slow walks. Balance exercises are especially important to reduce the risk of falls and injuries for older people; those with cancer that has spread to the bones and those who have osteoporosis, arthritis or peripheral neuropathy. Most likely you will be able to safely begin or maintain your own exercise program, but you may have better results with the help of an exercise specialist, physical therapist or exercise physiologist. Be sure to get your doctor's OK first and that the person working with you knows about your cancer diagnosis and any limitations you might have.

4)   Find a supportive cancer network

There are many support systems for persons living with cancer. Unlike most medical conditions, being affected by cancer means an overall transformation in your sense of yourself as a person with a body, mind and spirit. This has led to the development of the field of psycho-oncology.[26] One outcome is identifying *distress* as the "sixth vital sign" with the same importance as blood pressure, temperature, heart frequency, respiratory rate and pain. Another outcome is the formation of organizations, such as the American Psychosocial Oncology Society that offers a Helpline to connect cancer patients, their caregivers and advocacy organizations with psychiatrists, psychologists, nurses, social workers and counselors skilled in the management of cancer-related distress.

Five to Thrive® is a multi-media educational initiative created by Dr. Lise Alschuler and Karolyn A. Gazella that features an informational website, books, radio show, videos, social networks and a digital magazine.[27] They have a track record of employing an integrative approach to cancer prevention and treatment that can positively influence your health. Their Five To Thrive Plan is based upon five key bodily processes—immunity, inflammation, hormones, insulin sensitivity and digestion/detoxification.

A non-profit UK holistic cancer information organization www.canceractive.com includes the CANCERactive Patient Group (CAPG) – Run by Patients, for Patients. It offers you the opportunity to learn more about therapies that are specific for your form of cancer. For instance, you would find that cimetidine, an over-the-counter antacid, is beneficial in the treatment of colon cancer.

The American Association of Naturopathic Physicians can help you find a physician in your area to assist you in finding approaches tailored to your specific needs: http://www.naturopathic.org/.

Conclusion

Without question, there are things you can do to make the treatment of your cancer more effective. These complementary measures are based on what is known about how cancer cells form, as described in Chapter Five, and on the accumulating scientific evidence.

By becoming an expert in your particular form of cancer through your own research, you will find even more information about remedies and techniques that may be beneficial for you. Most importantly, you will find that you can become an active participant in your own cancer care. You even may be able to help your doctors with information they have not had time to collect. No practicing physician can keep up with all of the research and information that is pertinent to your situation. The trend in medical practice is to encourage patients to assume more responsibility in caring for their health, diseases and disabilities.

Cancer cries out for a holistic response, including fundamental changes in your lifestyle. All of us need to take greater personal responsibility for our health and wellbeing by making a commitment to physical exercise, stress relieving practices and eating unrefined, unprocessed, natural foods.

Chapter Twelve

Taking Charge of Being a Care Recipient or Caregiver

This chapter highlights special considerations for care recipients and caregivers living with cancer. It concludes with planning for your inevitable death that is important for everyone.

Just as care recipients have strong feelings about their situation, their caregivers are likely to have mixed emotions as well. The changes you go through in either role may well cause feelings of fear, anger, shame, frustration, helplessness, loneliness or depression. In order to ease your burdens, Fraser Health of British Columbia prepared a useful handbook for care recipients and for caregivers that I have drawn upon in this chapter.[1]

If You Are a Care Recipient

There's nothing good about being in a position where you must rely upon others to take care of you. Your symptoms and suffering are debilitating at least. Your dependency understandably can make you feel humiliated or even resentful. Seeing others who are comparatively healthy is not uplifting for you.

Elizabeth Kübler-Ross's 2005 book *On Grief and Grieving: Finding the Meaning of Grief Through the Five Stages of Loss* updates her ideas that have stood the test of time by outlining five possible stages in the way you may react to the grief precipitated by knowledge that you have a lethal form of cancer.[2] Awareness of these stages may help you and your caregivers understand emotions and behavior that can appear to be irrational but actually are natural responses to stress.

1 – <u>Denial</u> is a natural reluctance to accept the realities of your diagnosis.

2 – <u>Anger</u> at yourself and/or others. Why is this happening to me?

3 – <u>Bargaining</u> involves trying to make a deal with whatever forces you believe guide your destiny. If I do this, can I make it go away?

4 – <u>Depression</u> is the experience of sadness, regret, fear and uncertainty that shows you have begun to accept reality.

5 – <u>Acceptance</u> indicates that you have achieved emotional adjustment and objectivity. You may enter this stage a long time before the people you leave behind, who must pass through their own stages of dealing with grief.

More specifically in adjusting to your illness, you may:

- worry about becoming a burden for your spouse or children
- experience a sense of losing control over your life
- try to fight what is happening and try to hold on to the life you know
- fear that old friends will distance themselves from you
- experience sadness because of your changing self-image
- refuse to admit you need help or become demanding

At the same time, being a care receiver offers opportunities to model the qualities you admire in others: courage, optimism, bearing burdens, facing and dealing with reality and showing gratitude for the help you receive. It also gives you a chance to talk about your life, how you feel about death and your expectations about the future.

If You Are a Caregiver

"There are only four kinds of people in the world: those
who have been caregivers, those who are caregivers, those
who will be caregivers and those who need caregivers."
Former First Lady Rosalind Carter

You deserve special consideration as a caregiver. You need to know
how important you are not only to your loved one but to our society as
a whole. It's through your devotion and efforts that you make life better
and bearable for your loved one, but you can easily overlook how much
financial value you have for your own family and for society. Imagine what
it would be like to pay someone else to do what you do. You may know
already if you have found it necessary to shift caregiving to others in your
home or in a residential facility.

Caregivers often are reluctant to complain or to share their frustrations with others, even when those frustrations can be almost overwhelming. Those we care for obviously are grateful for what we do for them, but
they are suffering and frustrated to an extent that they may well be unable
to express gratitude and even may pose management problems for us.

Even under optimal circumstances people who love each other can
be annoying and even spiteful to each other. All of the ambivalence,
competitiveness and hostility that underlie normal, loving relationships
can pose significant problems for us. We can deny them. We can feel
guilty about them. We can lose our tempers. We can feel guilty. We can
even get depressed. All of these feelings lurk under the surface under the
best of circumstances. They are intensified when we are under stress or
are not feeling well for other reasons.

You may be a caregiver out of love or a sense of duty or both. When
you become a caregiver, you may take on roles that are very new to you.
You may have to learn new skills and do jobs that your spouse took care
of before, such as doing the housework, paying the bills or driving the car.

The daily wear and tear of providing care can test even the most patient and determined caregiver, especially when there are added demands,

such as when a loved one has dementia, is awake at night or is depressed and difficult to motivate. You also may have to help with personal tasks that are not the usual role of a spouse, such as toileting and bathing.

Many caregivers have said that the most stressful part of caregiving is emotional. You may find it hard to deal with some of your natural feelings. Maybe you think some of them are not acceptable. One minute you're angry because your loved one has done something that is upsetting for you. The next minute you feel sorry because you know that action wasn't intentional.

Common feelings described by family caregivers during the caregiving journey are fear, anger, grief and guilt. Caregivers may fear that they won't be strong enough or brave enough to do what needs to be done to help their loved ones in the face of ongoing crises and day-to-day challenges. You may feel angry for being forced into a role that you don't feel comfortable with, for putting your own plans on hold and for the loss of control of so many aspects of your life. You may feel angry at family and friends who have conflicting ideas about what should or should not be done.

Anger also may come from a sense of helplessness at watching your loved one's health diminish and disintegrate before your eyes, no matter how much care you are providing. There also is grief, where you may not only mourn the loss of the person who once was physically healthy, but also the changes in your relationship as you have known it. Perhaps the most haunting feeling described by family caregivers is the sense of guilt they experience. They believe they could have done things differently in the past to change the outcome.

What's more, there's new knowledge that needs to be learned about the disease and its course. It can seem at times that you must possess extraordinary problem solving strengths, which feels even more impossible when you already are feeling stretched.

Even when treatment is working, there are ups and downs in the course of caregiving. The most important downer is when treatment is not working, and a decision needs to be made about entering hospice care and whether or not it should be at home or in a residential facility.

Fortunately, hospice care workers and volunteers are in a position to be helpful at that point and later.

Hospice Care

Nonprofit hospice care is the most widely available and trusted end-of-life care that focuses on making you comfortable.[3] The word palliative often is used to describe its purpose. A team of health care professionals and volunteers provides it. They give medical, psychological and spiritual support. Their goal is to help people who are dying have peace, comfort and dignity. They try to control pain and other symptoms so you can remain as alert and comfortable as possible. Hospice programs also provide services to support your family.

In order to be accepted in hospice care usually you are expected to live 6 months or less, although there is considerable flexibility for accommodating each situation. Hospice care can take place

- At home
- At a hospice center
- In a hospital
- In a skilled nursing facility

If hospice care is received at home, you have assistance that eases your burden and gives you more freedom to pursue your interests away from home. If hospice care is received at a facility, the responsibilities of home care are relieved, but considerations about when and how often to visit arise. A new form of responsibility arises. On one hand, you have more freedom. On the other hand, the question arises as to how much time you should spend with your loved one in the facility. This is a time when all of the aforementioned underlying feelings can surface. Your visits can be determined by your needs more easily if your loved one has dementia and does not recognize you.

Caregiver-Care Receiver Understanding

In order to make the caregiver-care receiver relationship go as smoothly as possible, there are two general principles that need to be worked through between caregiver and care receiver...almost like a contract. The first is to establish an open line of communication in which each person feels free to express themselves. The second is to make explicit agreements.

Feeling free to express yourself is a vital foundation for working out agreements about the caregiving relationship. This means being able to ask for help, to complain, to express your frustrations and to lose your temper...for both of you. This freedom will prevent bottling up feelings that can be buried and indirectly affect both of you in ways that may not be recognized. For example, buried anger can lead to forgetting medications or feeling depressed. That buried anger also can explode irrationally. So agreeing to feel free to openly express bad feelings can give each of you space to be yourself and to understand and forgive each other. It also gives you space to be aware of the impact of your behavior on the other person and thereby more considerate of each other's perspective.

Caregivers inevitably feel guilt for a variety of reasons and to the extent possible do restrain themselves from expressing their negative feelings and adding to the burdens of their loved ones. The most common are related to feeling better off than your loved one and that there were some things you should have done or should not have done. The following up-front agreements about specific circumstances of caregiving are helpful in minimizing guilt:

- when I need to be away from home
- when we need to talk about something else
- when I need to be alone
- how much can the recipient be expected to do alone
- what I need to do for myself so that I can care for you

In spite of its downside, caregiving is the ultimate expression of love for another person. The experience provides an opportunity for intimate interactions that get to the heart of what life and death are all about. It offers opportunities for reflecting on the past, enjoying pleasurable moments in the present and planning realistically for the future. For caregivers and care recipients who are so inclined, it's a time for writing a memoir and assembling information and photographs about your family. It's a time to share memories and feelings.

The National Cancer Institute and the American Cancer Society provide more detailed information about caregiving on their web sites.[4]

Living Your Spiritual Life

> It is not you who are mortal, but only this body ... the
> spirit is your true self, not that physical figure.
> Cicero, *Tusculan Disputations*

Each one of us has a unique way of experiencing our spiritual lives, both knowingly and unknowingly. We may be devout members of religious organizations. We may participate regularly in meditation, yoga, tai chi, qigong or group activities. We may have our own unique ways of handling our attitudes toward our existence and health. Whatever our beliefs about life and death are, we are better-served by viewing our deaths as spiritual rather than as medical events.

If we have not worked out some ways to understand the meaning and purpose of our lives and to manage our feelings and health already, facing the end of our lives or the lives of loved ones brings us into situations in which we need to draw upon stress and anxiety relieving practices. This section is devoted to ways to do so based on neuroscience and meditation practices.

For many of us, various forms of prayer in the context of our religious faiths can be relied upon. Prayer is the most effective when it involves some form of intimacy with a superior power so that you feel deeply involved in the process rather than just reciting words.

For all of us, there are effective forms of meditation that can be relied upon for in-the-moment and enduring emotional and thoughtful refreshment. The key to all of them is coming into contact with your spiritual essence. In the language of neuroscience this means your conscious experience of the activities of your lower and higher brain centers, which in simplified terms includes your "*me*" (bodily sensations), your "*myself*" (your mind and its thoughts) and your "*I*" (your awareness of your body, mind and existence as a purposeful human being...your spirit).

*   "Me" = your body
*   "myself" = your mind
*   "I" = your spirit or soul

When we speak the word I, it's simply the personal pronoun we use to express our wishes, thoughts and feelings. In fact, the conscious awareness of your "*I*" of what you are saying follows your thoughts and words. "The thought just occurred to me" is an example of how your mind's words and thoughts are observed by your "*I*". Unconscious processes of your mind work behind the scenes to generate your thoughts and speech just as they do to create your emotions. How many times have you been surprised by what you have said...or wished you had not said? There are times when you consciously think about what you are going to say, but most of the time the words from your mind just come out directly as speech.

Your consciousness actually is just brain-wide broadcasting of information that is in your "global workspace"—a dense network of interconnected prefrontal and parietal brain regions.[5] Your "I" is more than consciousness. At any one time, you can only be conscious of a fragment of your brain activity within the limits of a single item or event although your "I" can take charge and quickly shift things into and out of your consciousness. So your "I" really is more than consciousness. There is a phantom in your head...your spirit or soul, or more technically an epiphenomenon of your brain like the electrical energy picked up by electroencephalographic electrodes placed on your scalp at any time.

When your "*I*" and my "*I*" connect, we have the sense that we are "*we*". This is most obvious when we make eye ("*I*") contact with each other. You usually can tell the difference between what it feels like when you are in genuine communication with another person and when you are not.

In one sense, it may be troubling to realize that you are at the mercy of your "*me*" and your "*myself*". In another sense, it is reassuring to know that they are just parts of your whole being and actually can be perceived, corrected and controlled by your "*I*".

The Detachment Exercise is an easily used form of meditation that permits you to clearly distinguish between your "*me*", your "*myself*" and your "*I*". This exercise is a way of knowing and understanding yourself and thereby is empowering.

The Detachment Exercise

The purpose of the detachment exercise is to detach your consciousness from the outer world, from your body and from your mind. It moves your attention beyond the vague images you see when you close your eyes and the background sounds that you hear when you are in quiet surroundings.[6]

You can detach from your surroundings, body and mind by assuming a comfortable sitting posture, closing your eyes and focusing on the moving in and out of air in your lungs for five to ten natural breaths. Then say to yourself silently or out loud something like the following slowly:

> "I have a body." Repeat "I can feel my body" until you can feel your body from your head to your toes. Then say, "My body can be tired or rested, sick or healthy, but I am more than my body. I have emotions that swing from love to hatred, from calm to anger and from joy to sorrow. I can observe these changes in my emotions. I have emotions, but I am not my emotions. I can respond or not respond to them."

Next, "I have a mind. I have thoughts and memories. My mind can think about my life, what I have done and what I want to do. I am using my mind now as I am speaking these words. I have a mind, but I am more than my mind."

Next, "I am observing my body- my "*me*". I am observing my mind- my "*myself*". I am "*I*" observing these things. My "*I*" is my spirit. My "*I*" is the tip of my true self."

Finally, while aware of being in your "*I*", your "*I*" can use your mind to evaluate your feelings and to discover what you really want to know or to do now.

With a little practice, you will be able to detach from any immediate situation and enter your "*I*" state. For example, at a red traffic light, you can detach and let your mind and feelings roam while waiting for it to turn green. When waiting for something to end or to happen, you can detach and enter your calm, creative "*I*" rather than turn on an externally stimulating electronic device. Your "*I*" is your best friend because it is your true self...your spirit.

More to the point, you can let your "*I*" perceive and guide your life by becoming aware of differences between the desires of your "*me*", the conflicting thoughts of your "*myself*" and the values of your "*I*".

You can tailor this exercise to fit your needs and circumstances. Some people find that just observing their breathing is enough to enter a completely relaxed state. Others find that focusing their "*I*" on an unsettling issue leads to its resolution. Others use this exercise as a setting for their prayer lives.

Discovering that you have an "*I*"...a spirit...really is empowering. Your spirit is the tip of your true self that can become consciously aware of how the social roles you play in life create *adaptive selves* (also called *false selves*) appropriate to those roles. Underneath them all is your "*I*"—your spirit and source of meaning and purpose in life.

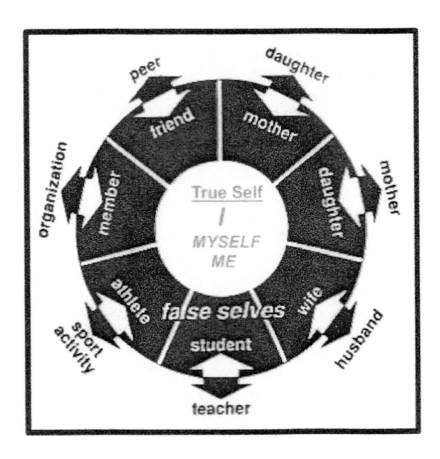

This diagram illustrates the *false selves*, the *true self*, the *I*, the *me* and the *myself* of a married woman with children in the context of her key social roles.

<u>Examples of Helpful Principles for Living</u>

<u>Prayer of St. Francis of Assissi</u>
Lord, make me an instrument of your peace.
Where there is hatred, let me sow love;
where there is injury, pardon;
where there is doubt, faith;
where there is despair, hope;
where there is darkness, light;
where there is sadness, joy.

Grant that I may not seek to be consoled but to console;
not to be understood but to understand;
not to be loved but to love.

For it is in giving that we receive;
it is in pardoning that we are pardoned;
and it is in dying that we are born to eternal life.

<u>Tao Te Ching</u>
Can you coax your mind from its wandering
and keep to the original oneness?
Can you let your body become
supple as a newborn child's?
Can you cleanse your inner vision
until you see nothing but the light?
Can you love people and lead them
without imposing your will?
Can you deal with the most vital matters
by letting events take their course?
Can you step back from your own mind
and thus understand all things?

Giving birth and nourishing,
having without possessing,
acting with no expectations,
leading and not trying to control:
these are the supreme virtues.

The Spacious Soul
Richard Rohr[7]

There is something in you that is not touched by coming
and going, by up and down, by for or against, by the
raucous teams of totally right or totally wrong. There is
a part of you that is patient with both goodness and evil
to gradually show themselves. There is a part of you that
does not rush to judgment. Rather, it stands as vigilant
and patient in the tragic gap that almost every moment
offers. It is a riverbed of mercy. It is vast, silent, restful,
and resourceful, and it receives and also lets go of all the
comings and goes. *It is awarenesss itself* (as opposed to
judgment itself) and awareness is not as such "thinking."
It is your True Self.

And you know what? Your soul is much larger than you!
You are just along for the ride. When you learn to live
there, you live with everyone and everything else too.
Any language of exclusion or superiority makes no sense
to you. Inside your True Self, you know you are not
alone, and you foundationally "belong" to the Universe.
You no longer have to work to feel important. You are
intrinsically important.

The 23rd Psalm

The Lord is my Shepherd; I shall not want.
He maketh me to lie down in green pastures:
He leadeth me beside the still waters.
He restoreth my soul:
He leadeth me in the paths of righteousness for His name' sake.

Yea, though I walk through the valley of the shadow of death,
I will fear no evil: For thou art with me;
Thy rod and thy staff, they comfort me.
Thou preparest a table before me in the presence of mine enemies;
Thou annointest my head with oil; My cup runneth over.

Surely goodness and mercy shall follow me all the days of my life,
and I will dwell in the House of the Lord forever.

Mindfulness Based Stress Reduction (MBSR)

If you want to more fully pursue stress relieving practices beyond or instead of yoga and other popular techniques, you can draw upon a growing literature and training programs devoted to mindfulness. MBSR was developed in 1979 by Jon Kabat-Zinn, an MIT-educated scientist. It's based on the principle that your attention is like a muscle. As with any muscle, it makes sense to exercise it through meditation to strengthen it. Even more to the point, exercising your power of attention develops stress-relieving qualities in your brain.

Kabat-Zinn has spawned a national movement devoted to adapting the principles and techniques described in his book *Full Catastrophe Living* to the needs of people in a variety of circumstances, ranging from improving work performance to relieving the pain and discomforts experienced by persons living with cancer.[8]

Neuroscientists have shown that meditation and rigorous mindfulness training can lower stress (cortisol levels and blood pressure) and even have an impact on the structure of the brain itself. Richard Davidson, founder and chair of the Center for Investigating Healthy Minds at the University of Wisconsin-Madison, noted that there are people who will not listen to someone in monks' robes, but they do pay attention to scientific evidence that mindfulness training works.[9] By 2012, 477 scientific journal articles had been published about mindfulness.[10]

Congressman Tim Ryan's personal experience bolstered by the empirical evidence led him to write *A Mindful Nation* in 2012 to promote teaching mindfulness in schools and more broadly in our society.[11]

Most Americans Do Not Die Well

If you are living with cancer and even if you are not, I hope that you are ready to think about the full course of your life, including the time in which you will die. I say this because our society does not handle death well. We seldom talk about it, and, when we do, we talk in abstract terms about whatever concept we have about what happens when we die. We do not see preparing for dying as a part of realistic living.

If you have been confronted with the diagnosis of cancer, you may have felt panic or at least worry about what is going to happen in the future. If you have not yet discovered that you have cancer, it still is worthwhile to think about what your reaction will be when you do know that you are dying from any cause. Hoping that you will die suddenly and not need to think about it is not the way it goes for the vast majority of us.

Research shows that most Americans do not die well, which is to say they do not die the way they say they want to—at home surrounded by the people who love them. According to data from Medicare, only a third of patients die this way.[12] More than 50 percent spend their final days in hospitals, often in intensive care units (ICUs) tethered to machines and feeding tubes or in nursing homes. The National Hospice and Palliative Care Organization estimates about 41 percent of hospice deaths occur at home.

Patients and families often pay a high price for difficult and prolonged deaths psychologically and economically. The Dartmouth Atlas Project, which gathers and analyzes health care data, found that 17 percent of

Medicare's $550 billion annual budget is spent on patients' last six months of life.[13] "We haven't bent the cost curve on end-of-life care," said Dr. David C. Goodman, a senior researcher for the project.

The amount spent on intensive care is climbing. Between 2007 and 2010, Medicare spending on patients in the last two years of their lives jumped 13 percent to nearly $70,000 per patient. The evidence is clear, Dr. Goodman said, that things could change if doctors "respect patient preferences and provide fair information about their prognosis and treatment choices."

There is a societal and professional reluctance to talk about death because it generally is regarded as a painful subject. Doctors basically are dedicated to improving and saving lives, not how lives end. In his book *Death Foretold*, Nicholas A. Christakis, a Yale sociologist, writes that few physicians offer patients a prognosis, and when they do, they do not do a good job.[14] Predictions, he argues, are often overly optimistic, with doctors being accurate just 20 percent of the time.

Without some basic understanding of the road ahead of them, Dr. Anthony L. Back, a University of Washington professor and palliative care specialist, said even sophisticated patients could end up where they least want to be: in an ICU. "They haven't realized the implications of saying: 'Yeah, I'll have that one more chemotherapy,'" Dr. Back said to Dan Gorenstein for his *The New York Times* article How Doctors Die: Showing Others the Way.[15]

Dr. Joan Teno, an internist and a professor of medicine at Brown University, told Gorenstein that people often avoid the difficult conversations they need to have together and with doctors about the emotional side of dying. "We pay for another day in an ICU," she said. "But we don't pay doctors to help patients think about their goals and values and then develop a plan."

On the positive side, the end-of-life choices Americans make are slowly shifting. Medicare figures show that there has been a modest increase in hospice care. At the same time, palliative care is being embraced on a broad scale, with most large hospitals offering such services.

There also is movement to talk about end of life plans as described in Chapter Three. For example, deathoverdinner.org, a website to help people hold end-of-life discussions, was started in 2013. The project's founder, Michael Hebb, said more than 1,000 dinner parties have been held, including some at nursing homes. The web site has gathered dozens of medical and wellness leaders to cast an unflinching eye at the end of life and has created an uplifting interactive adventure that transforms this difficult conversation into one of deep engagement.

A literature is growing on "dying well".[16] There even is a group discussion guide for Dr. Ira Byock's book, *Dying Well*. The basic themes are thinking about the way you would like to die and taking steps to try to ensure that your wishes are fulfilled. There are a number of books designed to help you plan wisely and effectively, such as *The End of Life Advisor* by nurses Susan Dolan and Audrey Vizzard.[17] In her book *Guide to the Great Beyond*, the *New York Times* health columnist Jane Brody has written an engaging and comprehensive book that aims to help you and your loved ones prepare, medically, legally and emotionally for the end of life.[18]

On September 18, 2007, Carnegie Mellon professor Randy Pausch delivered a one-of-a-kind last lecture "Really Achieving Your Childhood Dreams" that made the world stop and pay attention.[19] It became an Internet sensation viewed by millions, an international media story and a best-selling book that has been published in more than 35 languages.

In a vivid portrayal of his own life experience, Pausch offers advice in his book on how to get the most out of life. He discusses finding a happy medium between denial and being overwhelmed by cancer. He also states that he would rather die from cancer than be hit by a bus, because if he were hit by a bus, he would not have had the time he spent with his family nor the opportunity to prepare them for his death. On July 25, 2008, Diane Sawyer announced on Good Morning America that Pausch died of pancreatic cancer.

<u>Examples of Dying Well</u>

When it comes to dying, doctors and professors ultimately are no different from everyone else, and their emotional and physical struggles are surely every bit as wrenching. But physicians have a clear advantage over many of us. They have seen death up close. They understand their choices, and they usually know how to access the best that health care has to offer.

Dr. Elizabeth McKinley.

Dr. Elizabeth McKinley, a 53-year-old internist from Cleveland, battled breast cancer for 17 years.[20] In the spring of 2013, after Dr. McKinley's cancer found its way into her liver and lungs and the tissue surrounding her brain, she was told she had two options. "You can put chemotherapy directly into your brain, or total brain radiation," she recalled from her home in suburban Cleveland. "I'm looking at these drugs head-on and either one would change me significantly. I didn't want that." She also did not want to endure the side effects of radiation.

What Dr. McKinley wanted was time with her husband—a radiologist—and their two college-age children and another summer to soak her feet in the Atlantic Ocean. But most of all, she wanted "a little more time being me and not being somebody else." So, she turned down more treatment and began hospice care, the point at which the medical fight to extend life gives way to creating the best quality of life for the time that is left.

Dr. Robert Gilkeson, Dr. McKinley's husband, remembers his mother-in-law being unable to comprehend her daughter's decision. "'Isn't there some treatment we could do here?' she pleaded with me," he recalled. "I almost had to bite my tongue, so I didn't say, 'Do you have any idea how much disease your daughter has?'" Dr. McKinley and her husband were looking at her disease as doctors, who know the limits of medicine; her mother was looking at her daughter's cancer as a mother, clinging to the promise of medical treatment as limitless. Dr. McKinley died November 9, 2013, at home, where she wanted to be.

Dr. Sherwin Nuland

Author of the best-selling and award winning book *How We Die, Reflections on Life's Final Chapter* that has a study guide, surgeon Sherwin Nuland reiterated that life is finite.[21] He said that death—the coming end—is what gives life its meaning. It's what makes every living moment priceless. There's no time to procrastinate. There's no fountain of youth. This is it. Make the best of it.

Nuland's book portrays in unflinching detail how death occurs. He concluded that the idea of death with dignity was largely a fiction, unobtainable by most people. Instead, most people suffer interminably, often having the process prolonged through aggressive treatment by physicians and hospitals. Humiliation and lack of control, he said, are the fates of most.

Still, Nuland said that we can exert some control. By working closely with our medical team and circle of family and friends, we can do much to choose how we go out—opting for quality of life rather than one more heroic attempt to defeat the forces of illness and decay. And, even if we are wracked with pain or lost in a coma, we will find a "good death" if what has proceeded it has been a good life. The dignity that we seek in dying must be found in the dignity with which we have lived our lives."

Nuland died on March 3, 2014, of prostate cancer. He told his daughter Amelia, "I'm not scared of dying, but I've built such a beautiful life, and I'm not ready to leave it."

Professor Susan Gubar

Susan Gubar, Professor Emerita of English and Women's Studies at Indiana University, wrote about her encounter with ovarian cancer in *The New York Times* as follows.[22]

This year, 2013, was supposed to be the year of my death. When diagnosed in 2008, I was informed that I had three to five years left. Because of a clinical trial, I am living on borrowed time, which is experienced as a daily marvel. I realize, of course, that the trial extending my life will not cure me, that recurrence will probably be inevitable, along with palliative end-of-life care. Yet it is precisely this realization that intensifies my gratitude for being able to attend family gatherings at momentous events like a wedding, a birthday or a holiday during a succession of pain-free months.

I have been kept alive by my family, the clinical trial, the support group, and by Tara Parker-Pope, who encouraged me to embark on the Living with Cancer series of essays at just the moment I was accepted into the clinical trial. Lest you judge me daft for ranking a blog among my life-support systems, let me explain that writing these columns and reading your comments—which would never have happened without cancer and without the models provided by the other *The New York Times* writers Dana Jennings and Suleika Jaouad—have buoyed me up and cast me down and kept me thoroughly absorbed every day this year, engaged in what feels like a virtual community.

How can I refuse to grant cancer a positive role in my life, given these substantial rewards? Obstinate, I can and do.

For it is not cancer but rather a heightened sense of impending mortality that bestows these gifts, along with an appreciation of ongoing life never before lived, never again to be lived. Such awareness of embracing the impermanence and unpredictability of life and of those in our lives also sparks the urgency of testimony.

A famous line of poetry by Wallace Stevens—"Death is the mother of beauty."—comes into focus in a new way.

Only when we realize not that the other guy is going to die but that I am going to die do we see the beauty of transient existence and the beauty of trying to engage with its every facet, even the most fraught. The exaltation, the sheer pleasure of having been alive, of being alive, catches in the throat, brims tears in the eyes, for which we can only be glad. As for those cherished: no words are commensurate, just a delicate treasuring.

The Ways Children Experience Grief

The ways children express grief are usually different from the way adults express it.[23] Children are not always able to use words to express their feelings. Instead, they often express them through their behavior. Even children who are able to express themselves verbally may not always be able to express the many, sometimes conflicting, emotions they have. Children may:

+ Become very quiet, very talkative or overactive.
+ Have temper tantrums, angry outbursts or refuse to obey adults.
+ Have difficulty getting along with other children.
+ Return to younger behaviors, such as wetting the bed after they have been dry for months or years.
+ Cling to adults and want extra time and attention.
+ Have difficulty completing school work. Their grades may drop.

How children express grief usually depends on how they perceive the loss. Each child's perception of loss varies according to age and emotional development. In general:

+ Children younger than age 2 cannot understand the meaning of losses such as death of a family member. When a loss occurs, they know that something is different, but they do not know what it is. Because they are sensitive to the feelings of adults, they may become more fussy than usual.

- Children between the ages of 3 and 6 often think that any major change in their lives is a result of their actions or wishes. This is called magical thinking. These children often feel responsible for any loss that occurs. If they see a loss as a threat, they may think that they are being punished for something. If people leave them (such as in divorce), they may feel abandoned and scared. These children may react to loss by being afraid to be alone or to leave the people they love. They may not want to sleep alone at night and may refuse to go to day care or school. Other ways that children this age may express feelings of grief are by developing eating, sleeping or toileting problems.

- Children between the ages of 6 and 10 do not always fully understand events that occur in their lives. They may understand only part of what is going on around them, and they may invent conclusions or draw the wrong conclusions about things they do not understand, resulting in misconceptions about what is happening. They may develop fears, such as fear of death.

- Children between the ages of 10 and 12 start to understand loss (including death) the way adults do. They see death as permanent and irreversible. They are curious about what and how things happen. For example, if they have been affected by a hurricane, they may want to learn how hurricanes develop. If a person close to them dies, they may want to know how bodies are prepared after death, what the rites and rituals of burial mean and what happens to a person after he or she dies.

Resources to help you identify symptoms of severe stress and grief reactions in children and youth are available at the National Association of School Psychologist's website.[24]

Compassion and Choices

Compassion & Choices is the leading nonprofit organization committed to helping everyone have the best end of life experience possible by advocacy for "death with dignity" laws or judicial decisions permitting them, such as exist in Oregon, Washington, Montana, Vermont and New Mexico.[25] These laws allow mentally competent, terminally-ill adults to voluntarily request and receive a prescription medication to hasten their death.

In a landmark decision that terminally ill, mentally competent patients have a fundamental right to aid in dying under the substantive due process clause of the New Mexico State Constitution, New Mexico Second Judicial District Judge Nan Nash set forth a model rationale for death with dignity public policies on January 13, 2014:

> This Court cannot envision a right more fundamental, more private or more integral to the liberty, safety and happiness of a New Mexican than the right of a competent, terminally ill patient to choose aid in dying. If decisions made in the shadow of one's imminent death regarding how they and their loved ones will face that death are not fundamental and at the core of these constitutional guarantees, than what decisions are? ... The Court therefore declares that the liberty, safety and happiness interest of a competent, terminally ill patient to choose aid in dying is a fundamental right under our New Mexico Constitution.

Compassion and Choices also offers free counseling by telephone or the internet. It works across the nation to protect and expand options at the end of life. For over thirty years it has worked to reduce people's suffering and given them some control in their final days—even when injury or illness takes away their ability to communicate verbally. Compassion and Choices offers expertise in what it takes to die well. It provides information about ways in which to plan more specifically for your own dying process.

Additional Resources

For those who are attracted to the writings of theologian Paul Tillich, his classic book *The Shaking of the Foundations* shows how during times of suffering people can discover that they are not what they appear to be. Suffering reveals deeper levels of life's true meaning.[26]

Pastor Doug Manning's work in grief counseling was influenced by a couple from his church who lost a young daughter from a simple case of the croup. The mother was distraught and crying in the hospital room. The doctor and her husband were trying to calm her when she looked up and said, "Don't take my grief away from me. I deserve it and I am going to have it." He found that to be one of the most profound statements about what people in grief need, and this became the title of his book *Don't Take My Grief Away from Me.*[27]

Dr. Bernie Siegel shares the inspiring stories of people who have experienced cancer and found deeper faith, hope, joy and healing through the process in his book *Faith, Hope and Healing: Inspiring Lessons Learned from People Living with Cancer.*[28]

In his book *Anticancer: A New Way of Life*, Dr. David Servan-Scheiber drew upon his own experience with cancer and shared vivid descriptions of how to maintain an optimal mind-body balance through sickness and health by reducing your exposure to harmful toxins, maintaining a healthy diet and managing stress.[29]

Conclusion

Caregivers and care receivers have opportunities for intimate interactions and personal growth in the face of the challenges posed by debilitating illnesses. Facing the end of our lives challenges all of us to think about the meaning and purpose of life. Fortunately, there is a wealth of information, practices and organizations to help us handle the frustrations and responsibilities involved in taking charge of our lives with cancer.

Our society does not handle death well. As individuals, we do not see preparing for dying as a part of living and experiencing death as a spiritual rather than as a medical event. Still, an unappreciated part of living is thinking about what your reaction will be when you know that you are dying from cancer or from any other cause and planning for that certainty.

Hospice Care directly supports patients and their caregivers through a team-oriented group of specially trained professionals and volunteers and is available throughout the United States. Compassion & Choices offers free counseling, resource planning, referrals and guidance across the nation to protect and expand options at the end of life.

Chapter Thirteen

Where Are We Now?

This chapter summarizes the analyses by key organizations and individuals of the present state of the cancer field.

Michael P. Link, M.D., Past President of the American Society of Clinical Oncology (ASCO), said in 2013 that the pace of discovery about cancer remains exciting, but our capacity to deliver high-quality cancer care is being challenged as never before.[1]

Cancer Survival

The data on cancer survival can be interpreted either positively or negatively depending upon the agenda of the reporter. For example, in 2011 the Centers for Disease Control (CDC) painted a rosy picture in comparison to the ASCO *Accelerating Progress in Cancer* report in the same year.[2] The CDC stated that "as a result of advances in early detection and treatment, cancer has become a curable disease for some and a chronic illness for others." It went on to say that persons living with a history of cancer are now described as cancer survivors rather than cancer victims.

Although from 1971 to 2012, the number of people living with cancer in the United States increased from 3.0 million to 13.7 million, the annual cancer death rate has dropped 18% since the early 1990s, reversing decades of increases. The CDC said that this downturn in cancer death rates resulted mostly from reductions in tobacco use, increased screening allowing early detection of several cancers and modest to large improvements in the treatment of specific cancers.

In contrast, Clifton Leaf pointed out that, although the standardized death rate for cancer in America has fallen, the total number of cancer deaths in the country has risen by 74% since 1970.[3] That difference is explained by a growing and aging population, but it stands in contrast to the number of deaths from heart disease also sensitive to a growing and aging population, which has fallen by 19% during the same time. The percentage of Americans dying from cancer is about the same as in 1970... and in 1950. Cancer is the leading cause of death in the world.

The CDC also said that more people are surviving longer with cancer than ever. In 1980, half of cancer patients survived five years or more after diagnosis. The figure has crept up to two-thirds today. Yet here, too, the complete picture is not encouraging. Survival gains for the more common forms of cancer usually are measured in additional months of life, not years. The few dramatic increases in cure rates and patient longevity have come in a handful of less common malignancies—including Hodgkin's lymphoma, some leukemias, carcinomas of the thyroid and testes and most childhood cancers. Clifton Leaf adds, "It's worth noting that many of these successes came in the early days of the War on Cancer."

As an editor at *Fortune* magazine, Leaf became enthralled by the promise of Gleevec, an enzyme inhibitor that, since its release in 2001, has proven highly effective at battling chronic myeloid leukemia (CML). Many thought a new age was coming, in which the spread of cancer would be hindered by drugs that would be precision-targeted to block the replication of rogue cells. It seemed far better than indiscriminately killing both cancer and healthy cells, as chemotherapy had been doing for the past half-century.

But Gleevec is the exception, not the rule—and CML is a relatively simple cancer compared to solid-state tumors of the lung, colon, pancreas or breast. Once they metastasize, most cannot be cured. Many chemotherapeutic drugs are like pellets fired into cancer's flank. For example, a 2013 article in *The New York Times* hailed a new melanoma drug that increased the median survival rate by 16.8 months.[4] A 2013 editorial in *The Lancet*, the leading British medical journal, put the matter even more bluntly: "Has cancer medicine failed patients? In the words of cancer experts, the answer is yes."[5]

As of 2012, there were almost 13.7 million cancer survivors in the United States. By 2022, that number is expected to reach 18 million.[6] These patients will face higher risks of secondary cancers, cardiovascular disease, psychosocial issues and other health problems. "It's well established that treatment can induce a second malignancy or other late effects," said Lois Travis from the University of Rochester Medical Center in New York, who noted that the increasing number of cancer survivors also is a significant driver of health-care costs. Leslie Robison of St. Jude Children's Research Hospital said pediatric cancer survivors are at an up to 15-fold increased risk of death from secondary cancer, as well as a significantly greater risk of organ dysfunction, psychosocial problems and dysfunctions of fertility and reproduction, compared with children who have not had cancer.

New drugs often are disappointing because of flawed models for drug development, success measured by tumor shrinkage and the focus on cancer cells to the near exclusion of what's happening in the body as a whole. All these failures come to a head in the clinical trial for Food and Drug Administration approval—a rigidly controlled, possibly four-phase system for testing new drugs and other medical procedures in humans. The process remains the only way to get from research to drug approval—and yet it is hard to find anyone in the cancer community who isn't frustrated by it. This focuses our attention on the national leader in cancer research funding...the National Cancer Institute.

Funding Priorities of the National Cancer Institute (NCI)

In order to get a handle on the funding priorities of NCI, I surveyed the 170 page 2012 NCI Funded Research Portfolio consisting of 8,543 projects and came up with the following results for projects funded in the following categories that pertain to how cancer cells form (neoplasia):[7]

+ Cancer Etiology: (estimated by combining categories)
  $100,000,000 (2% of total budget)

- Cancer Initiation: Alterations in Chromosomes; Oncogenes & Tumor Suppressor genes:
  $33,616,418 (0.6% of total budget)
- Cancer Cell Biology:
  $134,507,651 (3% of total budget)
- Immunology:
  $580,000,000 (11.4% of total budget); calculated for me by Ryan Gilbert, NCI Budget Analyst.[8]

I was able to identify only $848,124,069 in the NCI Funded Research Portfolio devoted to projects that clearly focused on neoplasia out of a total of $5,058,104,978. This amounts to 17% of the total expenditures. A more sophisticated and extensive analysis undoubtedly would yield a higher total, but it's still unlikely to be at a level that the public expects of NCI, namely that it should be in the forefront of the War on Cancer. The vast majority of NCI funding as gone to the support of cancer facilities not to research that would lead to effective treatments for cancer.

I then read NCI Director Harold Varmus' Professional Judgment Budget 2013.[9] Here is what Dr. Varmus said:

> Over the years, the Congress and the public have generously supported the NCI—and the NIH generally—with sustained budgetary increases. This was especially true for the NCI during the rapid expansion of its budget following the National Cancer Act of 1971 and for the NIH, including the NCI, during the five-year doubling of its budget, launched in 1998. Both of these eras of rapid growth were remarkably fruitful. The first launched the pursuit of cancer genes and the molecular basis of oncogenesis, laying the foundation for the transformation of clinical oncology that is now occurring. The latter accelerated the completion of the human genome project that now guides the study and control of all diseases, including cancers. Since 2003, however, the budgets of the NCI and the NIH have grown

minimally, with their buying power shrinking by about 20
percent as a consequence of inflation.

This decade-long hiatus in financial growth has come,
ironically, at a time of unmatched promise in the oncologi-
cal sciences and at a time when the world of cancer research
has expanded in talent, facilities, and ideas. Progress in
molecular biology, especially in the deciphering of cancer
genomes and the probing of the signaling pathways that
govern normal and malignant cell growth, has transformed
our ability to understand the broken parts of a cancer cell;
to develop new and more precise therapeutic strategies; to
begin to reformulate diagnostic categories; and to imagine screening for and prevention of some cancers in more
powerful ways. In just the past few years, NCI-supported
science has delivered a remarkable collection of genetic
information about several types of cancers, a number of
new targeted therapies for various cancers, compelling
examples of successful immunologically based-therapies,
persuasive evidence that radiographic screening can reduce lung cancer mortality, and many new observations
about the genesis of cancer cells, their development, their
behavior, and their micro-environment.

As an administrator of a federal agency, Dr. Varmus obviously
wanted to be as positive as possible, however, the 2013 National Cancer
Institute Provocative Questions initiative designed as a challenging
intellectual exercise for researchers to define and then solve the major
unsolved or neglected problems in oncology does not reflect his vision.[10]
Understandably, the priorities represented the areas of interest to the
persons who suggested the Questions. Out of 20 questions suggested as
appropriate for NCI funding in 2013 only 5 (underlined in table) were
targeted on projects that might yield new more effective treatments based
on the causes of cancer cell formation and growth.

National Cancer Institute: The "Provocative Questions" Initiative - 2013

Group A: Cancer Prevention and Risk

PQA - 1. *How do decision making processes influence habitual behaviors, and how can that knowledge be used to design strategies that lead to adoption and maintenance of behaviors that reduce cancer risk?*

PQA - 2. *How does the level, type, or duration of physical activity influence cancer risk and prognosis?*

PQA - 3. *What biological mechanisms influence susceptibility to cancer risk factors at various stages of life?*

PQA - 4. *For tumors that arise from a pre-malignant field, what properties of cells in this field can be used to design strategies to inhibit the development of future tumors?*

Group B: Mechanisms of Tumor Development or Recurrence

PQB - 1. *Why do second, independent cancers occur at higher rates in patients who have survived a primary cancer than in a cancer-naïve population?*

PQB - 2. *What molecular and cellular events in the tumor microenvironment (for example, the local immune response) determine if a tumor at the earliest stages of malignant transformation is eliminated, stimulated for further development, or made indolent?*

PQB - 3. *What mechanisms initiate or sustain cancer cachexia, and can we target them to extend lifespan and quality of life for cancer patients?*

PQB - 4. *What methods can be devised to characterize the functional state of individual cells within a solid tumor?*

Group C: Tumor Detection, Diagnosis, and Prognosis

PQC - 1. *What properties of pre-cancerous lesions or their microenvironment predict the likelihood of progression to malignant disease?*

PQC - 2. *What molecular or cellular events establish tumor dormancy after treatment and what leads to recurrence?*

PQC - 3. *How do variations in tumor-associated immune responses among patients from distinct well-defined populations, such as various racial/ethnic or age groups, contribute to differences in cancer outcomes?*

PQC - 4. *What in vivo imaging methods can be developed to portray the "cytotype" of a tumor — defined as the identity, quantity, and location of each of the different cell types that make up a tumor and its microenvironment?*

Group D: Cancer Therapy and Outcomes

PQD - 1. *What molecular properties make some cancers curable with conventional chemotherapy?*

PQD -2. *What features of standard-of-care therapies enhance or inhibit the efficacy of immunotherapy?*

PQD - 3. *Do tumors evolve common features that could act as new therapeutic targets when they metastasize to the same secondary site?*

PQD - 4. *What are the mechanistic bases for differences in cancer drug metabolism and toxicity at various stages of life?*

Group E: Clinical Effectiveness

PQE - 1. *What strategies optimize adoption and sustainability of guideline concordant cancer treatments in community settings?*

PQE - 2. *What care delivery models can be developed to transition cancer patients effectively from active therapy to end of life care?*

PQE - 3. *What methods and approaches induce physicians and health systems to abandon ineffective interventions or discourage adoption of unproven interventions?*

PQE - 4. *What are the best methods to identify and stratify subgroups of patients with particular co-morbidities who will benefit from defined cancer therapies?*

If the public, especially persons with cancer, had been asked for provocative questions, we would have simply said: find out what causes cancer and how to prevent, stop and reverse those causes. The lack of prioritizing this fundamental goal of curing cancer by the NCI is puzzling in the light of the importance of cancer as the number one cause of death in the world.

Hopefully Dr. Varmus' commitment to changing the conversation about cancer will fulfill the aim of the American Association of Clinical Oncology to vastly improve cancer research and care.

Turning the Tide on the War on Cancer

Clifton Leaf underscores the fact that for our nation finally to turn the tide in the War on Cancer, the cancer community must embrace a coordinated assault. Doctors and scientists now have enough knowledge to do what Sydney Farber hoped they might do 33 years ago: to work as an army, not as individuals fighting on their own. It isn't just the patients in the War on Cancer who need renewed hope. It is the foot soldiers as well.

The National Cancer Institute (NCI) can begin this transformation right away by changing the way it funds research. It can undo the culture created by separate grants focused on individual projects by shifting the balance of financing to favor cooperative projects focused on the big picture. The NCI already has such funding in place, for endeavors called Specialized Programs of Research Excellence (SPORE).[11] These grants bring together researchers from different disciplines to solve aspects of the cancer puzzle. Even so, funding for individual study awards accounts for a full quarter of the agency's budget and is more than 12 times the money spent on SPORE grants. In Leaf's words, "the agency needs to stop being an automatic teller machine for basic science and instead use the taxpayers' money to marshall a broad assault on this elusive killer—from figuring out how to stop metastasis in its tracks to coming up with testing models that better mimic human response."

Just as importantly, Leaf urges the cancer leadership, the Food and Drug Administration (FDA) and lawmakers to transform drug testing and approval into a process that delivers information on what's working and what's not to patients far faster. If the best hope to treat most cancer lies in using combinations of drugs, legal constraints will need to be removed to give drug companies incentives to work together in testing investigational compounds in shorter trials. These should be funded by the NCI in a process that's distinct from individual drug approval. One bonus for the companies could be: if joint activity showed marked improvement in survival, the FDA process could be jump-started.

"It's going to require a community conversation to facilitate this change," Eli Lilly's Executive Vice President of Drug Development Homer Pearce said to Leaf. "I think everyone believes that at the end of the day, cancer is going to be treated with multiple targeted agents—maybe in combination with traditional chemotherapy drugs, maybe not. Because that's where the biology is leading us, it's a future that we have to embrace—though it will definitely require different models of cooperation."

Third Rock Ventures is an example of the kind of firm that is using collaboration and integration in maximizing the effectiveness of investing in medical technology.[12] Instead of maximizing the separate profits of venture firms, payers, hospitals, insurers, and doctors this firm focuses on a single system view including as many parties as possible in planning and developing new products.

Leaf goes on to say that to find out which drugs truly have promise we need to do one thing more often: test them on people in less advanced stages of disease. The reason, once again, comes back to cancer's genetic instability—a progression that not only ravages the body but also riddles tumors with mutations. When cancer patients are in the end stage, drugs that might have a potent effect on newer cancers fail to show much progress at all. Our current crop of rules, however, pushes drug companies into a can't-win situation, where the only way out is incremental improvements to existing therapies. Drugs that might well help some cancer patients are now getting tossed by the wayside because they don't help the people they couldn't have helped in any case. This has to stop.

Dr. Link also asks how will we keep the pharmaceutical industry engaged in the development of new treatments when we are pursuing specific targets of interest in increasingly narrow populations with lower revenue prospects?

Conclusion

The data on cancer survival can be interpreted either positively or negatively depending upon the viewpoint of the reporter. Unfortunately, it is based on five-year survival rates that too often involve an impaired if not miserable quality of life. The bottom line is that cancer is the foremost cause of death in the world, and we are not winning the War on Cancer.

Clinicians and scientists now have enough knowledge to work as an army, not as individuals fighting on their own, which has been the dominant pattern. The National Cancer Institute is beginning this transformation by financing cooperative projects focused on the big picture.

In order to find out which drugs truly have promise they need to be tested on people in less advanced stages of disease. When cancer patients are in the end stage, drugs that might have had a potent effect on newer cancers fail to show much progress at all.

Public understanding of the situation and pressure for change is needed to point cancer research and care on the prevention, interruption and reversal of neoplasia.

Chapter Fourteen

Obstacles to Progress

The powerful ideological, conceptual, political and financial obstacles to altering the status quo in the cancer field are outlined.

Because of the potential devastating outcomes of most forms of cancer, emotions can get in the way of progress in cancer care. Some persons have a cancer phobia that complicates their lives and causes unnecessary worry. At the same time, there is a strong tendency to avoid facing the facts about cancer that can lead to the opposite—namely a denial of those facts.

One consequence is the general reluctance of doctors to confront patients with uncomfortable truths. They view themselves as having a responsibility to reduce anxiety and suffering. This leads them to stress positives rather than negatives.

As a result, as the American Society of Clinical Onocology (ASCO) points out, most cancer patients aren't informed about the facts regarding their prognoses. They're not told that initial positive responses to treatment don't mean that a cure is at hand. In fact, even the idea that there's a cure for cancer overlooks the fact that cancer cells are products of the underlying biological process neoplasia that reflects a failure of the body's immune system to do its job. The truth is that cancer remains poorly understood and managed, as the ASCO's 2011 *Accelerating Progress against Cancer* report reveals...uncertainty prevails.

Our forefathers dealt with uncertainty on a daily basis to a degree that we would find unfathomable today. The West was tamed without

GPS devices, cell phones, rescue helicopters or any of the technologies and services we now take for granted. Technology has improved our lives significantly, but it also has affected our ability to deal with uncertainty, both individually and as a society. We seem to be increasingly intolerant of uncertainty. We seem to believe that the unpredictable should be predicted, and, if bad things happen, someone is to be blamed. In fact, despite all our technology and advancements in knowledge, we still have limited control over what happens in our lives and in the world.

All of this sets the stage for contemporary professionals feeling the need to minimize the uncertainties and stress that arise when persons are informed that they have a life-threatening form of cancer. They also need to put a positive face on their efforts to help patients in order to sustain their own sense of usefulness and purpose in their work. It's not easy to spend every working day dealing with patients who are suffering and confronted with a limited life span. It takes courage and compassion, often flavored with an upbeat attitude, to work in the cancer field. Fortunately, there are positive outcomes that lead to expressions of gratitude from patients...and there are patients who are free of observable cancer for years.

In his 2011 ASCO Presidential Address, Dr. Michael Link noted that "As difficult as it is these days, I admit that I am willing to abide by the advice provided by Albert Einstein, a very wise scientist indeed: 'Not everything that can be counted counts.' The wonderful and unique relationship between oncologist and patient and what it provides to both patient and physician is valuable, even if that part of what we do is not always valued."[1]

Dr. Link noted that the current pace of discovery is exciting, but the capacity to deliver high-quality care is being challenged as never before. He said: "We have entered an era of medicine with growing emphasis on economics and quantitation: risk-benefit ratios, quality-adjusted life-years, numbers needed to treat, and more. And the increasingly mundane stuff that has intruded as a result of the 'businessification' of medicine as well: profit and loss; the economics of sustaining our practices; viewing physicians and patients as 'providers' and 'customers'; a sustainable growth rate; and the ever more pervasive relative value unit."

Dr. Link's point was made even more strongly by Dr. Otis Brawley, chief medical officer for the American Cancer Society, in his book *How We Do Harm: A Doctor Breaks Ranks about Being Sick in America*.[2] Dr. Brawley provides documentation that the American health system is fundamentally flawed. He concluded: "The system is not failing. It's functioning exactly as designed, with the greedy serving the gluttonous. While low-income Americans are denied adequate medical care, the wealthy also are poorly served, often paying for unneeded treatments that can have dangerous side effects."

In this context, people with cancer and the general public aren't served well by administrators, physicians, industries and organizations who point to increased five-year survival rates as indicating progress in the cancer field. Even the ASCO 2011 report *Accelerating Progress Against Cancer* presents a nuanced critical view of the current state of cancer that has unnecessarily taken the lives of millions of persons because of decades of misdirected and underfunded research.

The Failure to Act on the Causes of Cancer

In his book *Cancer Wars*, the historian Robert Proctor bluntly stated in 1995, "The causes of cancer are largely known—and have been for quite some time. Cancer is caused by chemicals in the air we breathe, the water we drink, and the food we eat."[3]

The epidemiologist Devra Davis, who was the first director of the Center for Environmental Oncology at the University of Pittsburgh Cancer Institute, went further in *The Secret History of the War on Cancer*, alleging that political inaction over environmental carcinogens has its roots in the influence of industrial chemical companies—both those that profit by making pesticides and other cancer causing chemicals and those that profit by making cancer drugs.[4] Depending on how you parse the notions of causes, fighting cancer means more environmental cleanup, green politics and dietary reform—all politically contentious issues.

Davis points out that the War on Cancer has focused far too much on treatment, and not enough on prevention. There's a lot of blame to go around, and Davis serves it up to the scientific community, the government, polluting industries and even cancer advocacy groups. For instance, in the late 1960s, three years after the Surgeon General declared that smoking causes cancer, the federal government spent $30 million of taxpayer money to create safer cigarettes, essentially doing the tobacco companies' research and development for them. Needless to say, this effort failed, but it succeeded in giving the tobacco companies cover by assuring smokers that a safer cigarette was just around the corner.

Davis argues that again and again from tobacco to benzene to asbestos the profit motive has trumped concerns about public health, delaying— sometimes for decades—the containment of avoidable hazards, such as air pollution. In this vein, the current "scientific debate" about global warming has been exploited by industries to promote the idea that there's really no need to worry about global warming, distracting the public from the fact that the pollution of our air cannot be questioned. This has led to reporting air quality as "good" when the pollution is only mild.

Davis reveals that one of the foremost epidemiologists of the 20th century was "on the take" from Monsanto to the tune of $1,500 a day. She also reminds us of the sites of former towns that have literally disappeared, like Times Beach, Missouri, which was declared a toxic waste site, incinerated and reduced to some grass and flowers— the only signs that anyone ever had lived there.

In 2003 Samuel S. Epstein, chairman of the Cancer Prevention Coalition, in "The Stop Cancer Before It Starts Campaign: How to Win the Losing War Against Cancer" called attention to the failure to warn the public of cancer risks from avoidable exposures to industrial carcinogens and ionizing radiation.[5] This is in striking contrast to the cancer establishment's stream of press releases, briefings and media reports proclaiming the latest advances in cancer screening, treatment and basic research. This relative silence about cancer prevention also violates the 1988 Amendments to the National Cancer Act that called for "an expanded and intensified research program for the prevention of cancer caused by occupational or environmental factors."

Institutional Finances

The "businessification" of medicine described by Dr. Link poses management advantages but clearly distorts the priorities of the health care system. This is nowhere more apparent than in the cancer field.

As an example, major academic medical centers in New York and around the country are spending heavily on genomic analysis equipment in what has become an "arms race" within the War on Cancer.[6] The investments are based on the belief that the medical establishment is moving toward the routine sequencing of every patient's genome in the quest for "precision medicine" based on the unique characteristics of each patient's genes.

At this point, scientists only have an imperfect understanding of how snippets of genetic material can determine a patient's chances of getting many diseases, especially more common ones. But by setting up the right infrastructure—collecting and sequencing patient DNA, identifying patients who could benefit from a particular drug and aggressively recruiting patients for trials—the academic medical centers hope to play a bigger role in the development of new drugs.

Mount Sinai's medical school has installed a new $3 million supercomputer that makes quick work of huge amounts of genetic and other biological information. Just a couple of miles away a competitor—NewYork-Presbyterian Hospital/Weill Cornell Medical Center—is building a $650 million research tower. Across the street is a newly completed $550 million tower housing labs for another competitor, Memorial Sloan-Kettering Cancer Center.

Dr. James M. Crawford, chair of pathology at Hofstra North Shore-LIJ School of Medicine, said his institution, a competitor in some ways with the Manhattan medical centers, was "quite literally on the fence" about whether to join this "arms race" or to "let more data emerge before we decide we are going to commit more resources to this."

In a similar vein, Congressional investigators from the Government Accountability Office said in a 2013 report that doctors who have a financial interest in radiation treatment centers are much more likely to prescribe such treatments for patients with prostate cancer.[7] The investigators said that Medicare patients often were unaware that their doctors stood to profit from the use of radiation therapy. Alternative treatments may be equally effective and are less expensive, the report said. In other recent studies, the auditors found a similar pattern when doctors owned laboratories and imaging centers that billed Medicare for CT scans and magnetic resonance imaging.

In his 1997 book *World Without Cancer*, G. Edward Griffin, film producer and author, revealed a shocking picture of how science has been subverted to protect entrenched commercial and political interests.[8] He contended that the answer is based upon the economic and power goals of those who control the medical/pharma establishment.

In *Overdosed America: The Broken Promise of American Medicine*, the physician John Abramson described in 2004 a profound shift that has taken place in the culture of American medicine.[9] Tests unlikely to improve patient care are being routinely ordered, and expensive drugs that had not been shown to be any more effective or safer than the older drugs they are replacing are being routinely prescribed.

Many patients are being drawn in by the growing number of drug ads and medical news stories. Patients are increasingly arriving for their medical visits with a firm idea of the outcome they want instead expectating that the best care would emerge from a discussion of their symptoms, concerns and examination and then mutual consideration of the options. An example is the recent emphasis on prescribing statin drugs to reduce the risk of heart disease and stroke by the American Heart Association and the American College of Cardiology, organizations heavily supported by drug industries.[10] This distracts people from the factors that undeniably reduce the risk of cardiovascular disease: healthy diets, exercise and avoiding smoking.

Gilbert Welch, a professor of medicine at the Dartmouth Institute for Health Policy and Clinical Practice, is an author of *Overdiagnosed: Making People Sick in the Pursuit of Health*.[11] The book outlines a complex web of factors that has created the phenomenon of overdiagnosis: 1) the popular media promotes fear of disease and perpetuates the myth that early, aggressive treatment is always best; 2) in an attempt to avoid lawsuits, doctors can leave no test undone and no abnormality overlooked and 3) profits are being made from screenings, medical procedures and pharmaceuticals. Revealing the social, medical and economic ramifications of a health-care system that overdiagnoses and overtreats patients, Dr. Welch makes a reasoned call for change that would save all of us pain, worry and money.

Complementary and Alternative Medicine

Complementary and alternative medicine (CAM), as defined by the National Center for Complementary and Alternative Medicine (NCCAM), constitute a group of medical and health care systems, practices and products that are not presently considered to be part of conventional medicine. Over half of all cancer patients use CAM therapies.[12] Complementary medicine is used together with conventional medicine. Alternative medicine is used in place of conventional medicine. Conventional medicine is practiced by holders of medical or osteopathy degrees and by health professionals who work with them, including physical therapists, psychologists and registered nurses. Other terms for conventional medicine include allopathy; Western, mainstream, orthodox and regular medicine; and biomedicine. Some conventional medical practitioners are also practitioners of CAM.

The National Center for Complementary and Alternative Medicine (NCCAM) is the federal government's lead agency for scientific research on CAM to explore complementary and alternative healing practices in the context of rigorous science, training CAM researchers and disseminating authoritative information to the public and professionals. NCCAM defines integrative medicine as treatment that combines conventional medicine with CAM therapies that have been reported to be safe and effective after being studied in patients. In practice, many CAM therapies used in along with conventional medicine have not yet been tested in this way.

The National Cancer Institute (NCI) and the Office of Cancer

Complementary and Alternative Medicine are sponsoring a number of clinical trials at medical centers to evaluate CAM therapies for cancer. Cancer patients using or considering complementary or alternative therapy should discuss this with their doctor or nurse, as they would any therapeutic approach. Some complementary and alternative therapies may interfere with, or may be harmful when used with, conventional treatment. It also is a good idea to become informed about a therapy, including whether the results of scientific studies support the claims that are made for it.

In his book *Do You Believe in Magic?* Dr. Paul A. Offit offers a parallel scathing exposé of the alternative medicine industry, revealing how even though some popular therapies are remarkably helpful possibly due to the placebo response, many of them are ineffective, expensive and even deadly.[13] He reveals how alternative medicine—an unregulated industry under no legal obligation to prove its claims or admit its risks—can actually be harmful to our health.

Offit points out that any therapy—alternative or conventional—should be scrutinized. He shows how some alternative medicine methods can do a great deal of good, in some cases exceeding therapies offered by conventional practitioners. Still, Offit cites the important dictum: there is really no such thing as "alternative" medicine, but only medicine that has been shown to work effectively and safely. If it hasn't been shown to be safe and effective, there's no point in calling any treatment "medicine".

A growing lobby of Complementary and Alternative Medicine providers want the government to require insurance providers to pay for treatments, regardless of whether or not they work.[14] The strategy is simple: require the government to fund any treatment that a patient wants as "patient choice."

In his book *Catastrophic Care*, David Goldhill points to the answer: design a fair system where everyone receives an adequate—and sufficient—amount of health care.[15] Better solutions to allocate our precious medical resources will be revealed after our nation ceases to regard health as a commodity and comes to understand the key principle that health care is a public good.

Problems with Research Reproducibility

The idea that experiments should be reproducible was the defining feature of science for Roger Bacon back in the 13th century and is the cornerstone of science today. Reasons for the lack of reproducibility include intentional fraud and misconduct, negligence, inadvertent errors, imperfectly designed experiments, the biases of the researchers and other uncontrollable variables.

Most importantly, the replication of published research is not a priority for scientists and journal editors today. Scientific honors go to those who publish new results not to those who confirm or challenge existing results. This situation spawned The Reproducibility Project as an empirical effort to estimate the reproducibility of a sample of studies from the psychological scientific literature.[16] The project is a large-scale, open collaboration currently involving more than 150 scientists from around the world. It's sponsored by the Center for Open Science, a non-profit organization based in Charlottesville, Virginia, and dedicated to improving the alignment between scientific values and scientific practices to improve the accumulation and application of knowledge.

Jalees Rehman, an Associate Professor of Medicine and Pharmacology at the University of Illinois at Chicago, notes that the cancer researchers Glenn Begley and Lee Ellis made a rather remarkable claim last year.[17] They revealed that scientists at the biotechnology company Amgen were unable to replicate the vast majority of published pre-clinical research studies. Only 6 out of 53 landmark cancer studies could be replicated, a dismal success rate of 11 percent.

The claims of low reproducibility made by Begley and Ellis referred to pre-clinical science. The lack of reproducibility in pre-clinical cancer research has a significance that reaches far beyond just cancer research. If only 11 percent of published landmark papers in cancer research are reproducible, questions are raised about publications in other areas of biological research.

Lee Ellis co-authored another paper to delve further into this question.[18] Only 17 percent of their colleagues responded to their anonymous survey, but the responses confirmed that reproducibility of papers in peer-reviewed scientific journals is a major problem. Two-thirds of the senior faculty respondents revealed they had been unable to replicate published findings, and the same was true for roughly half of the junior faculty members as well as trainees. What's more, Ellis affirmed that researchers are reluctant to try to replicate the work of others because academic and monetary rewards come from their own original work.

Scientists need to acknowledge that reproducibility is a major problem. Recent questions raised about the reproducibility of biological and medical research findings are forcing scientists to embark on a soul-searching mission...can they believe each other?

Feel-Good War on Breast Cancer

In a popular vein, Peggy Orenstein wrote a critical article in *The New York Times Magazine* titled "Feel-Good War on Breast Cancer."[19] She noted that, according to Robert Aronowitz, a professor of history and sociology of science at the University of Pennsylvania and the author of *Unnatural History: Breast Cancer and American Society*, physicians endorsed the idea of a War on Cancer partly out of wishful thinking, desperate to "do something" to stop a scourge against which they felt helpless. So in 1913, a group of them banded together, forming an organization (which eventually became the American Cancer Society) and alerting women in a precursor of today's mammography campaigns that surviving cancer was within their power. By the late 1930s, they had mobilized a successful "Women's Field Army" of more than 100,000 volunteers dressed in khaki who went door to door raising money for "the cause" and educating neighbors to seek immediate medical attention for "suspicious symptoms," like lumps or irregular bleeding.

The campaign worked—sort of. More people did go to their doctors. More cancers were detected, more operations were performed and more patients survived their initial treatments. But the rates of women dying of breast cancer hardly budged. That should have been a sign that some aspect of the early-detection theory was amiss. Instead, surgeons believed they just needed to find the disease even sooner.

Mammography promised to do just that. The first trials, begun in 1963, found that screening healthy women along with giving them clinical exams reduced breast-cancer death rates by about 25 percent. It seemed only logical that finding cancer earlier would yield even more impressive results if women underwent annual mammography. By the early 1980s, an estimated fewer than 20 percent of those eligible did. So Nancy Brinker founded the Komen foundation in 1982 to boost those numbers, convinced that early detection and awareness of breast cancer could have saved her sister, Susan, who died at the age of thirty-six. Three years later, National Breast Cancer Awareness Month was born. The khaki-clad "soldiers" of the 1930s were replaced by millions of pink-garbed racers "for the cure" as well as legions of pink consumer products: pink buckets of chicken, pink yogurt lids, pink vacuum cleaners and pink dog leashes.

Even as American women embraced mammography, researchers' understanding of breast cancer—including the role of early detection—was shifting. Breast cancer, it has become clear, does not always behave in a uniform way. It's not even one cancer. There're at least four genetically distinct breast cancers. They may have different causes and respond differently to treatment. Within those classifications, there're doubtless further distinctions—subtypes that may someday yield a wider variety of drugs that can isolate specific tumor characteristics and allow for more effective treatment. But that's still years away.

Gilbert Welch, a professor of medicine at the Dartmouth Institute for Health Policy and Clinical Practice and co-author of the 2012 *New England Journal of Medicine* study of screening-induced overtreatment, estimated that only 3 to 13 percent of women whose cancer was detected by mammograms actually benefited from the test.[20]

Despite the fact that Komen trademarked the phrase "race for the cure," Orenstein noted that only 16 percent of the $472 million raised in 2011 went toward research. At $75 million, that's still enough to give credence to the claim that Komen has been involved in every major breast-cancer breakthrough for the past 29 years. Still, the sum is dwarfed by the $397 million the foundation spent on administration, education, screening and other expenses. What's more, according to a *Fortune* magazine analysis, only an estimated .5 percent of all National Cancer Institute grants since 1972 focus on cancer metastasis.[21]

At the same time, the function of the pink-ribbon culture—and Komen in particular—has become less about eradicating breast cancer than self-perpetuation: maintaining the visibility of the disease and keeping the funds rolling in. "These campaigns all have a similar superficiality in terms of the response they require from the public," said Samantha King, associate professor of kinesiology and health at Queen's University in Ontario and author of *Pink Ribbons, Inc.: Breast Cancer and the Politics of Philanthropy.*[22] "They're divorced from any critique of health care policy or the politics of funding biomedical research. They reinforce a single-issue competitive model of fund-raising. And they whitewash illness: we're made 'aware' of a disease yet totally removed from the challenging and often devastating realities of its sufferers."

"It's tricky," Susan Love, a breast surgeon and president of the Dr. Susan Love Research Foundation, said to Ornstein. "Some young women get breast cancer, and you don't want them to ignore it, but educating kids earlier—that bothers me. Here you are, especially in high school or junior high, just getting to know your body. To do this search-and-destroy mission where your job is to find cancer that's lurking even though the chance is minuscule to none...it doesn't serve anyone. And I don't think it empowers girls. It scares them."

One hundred and eight American women die of breast cancer each day. Some can live for a decade or more with metastatic disease, but the median life span is 26 months. Scientific progress is erratic and unpredictable. "We are all floundering around in the dark," Peter B. Bach, director of the Center for Health Policy and Outcomes at Memorial Sloan-Kettering Cancer Center, told Ornstein. "The one thing I can tell you is some of that floundering has borne fruit. There are a few therapies—like tamoxifen and Herceptin—that target specific tumor characteristics and newer tests that estimate the chance of recurrence in estrogen-positive cancers, allowing lower-risk women to skip chemotherapy. That's not curing cancer," Bach said, "but it's progress. And yes, it's slow."

It has been four decades since the former first lady Betty Ford went public with her breast-cancer diagnosis, shattering the stigma of the disease. It has been three decades since the founding of Komen. Two decades since the introduction of the pink ribbon. Yet Orenstein points out that all that well-meaning awareness has ultimately made women less conscious of the facts by obscuring the limits of screening, conflating risk with disease, compromising our decisions about health care and celebrating "cancer survivors" who may have never required treatment.

Perspectives on Cancer

Looking for fresh insights into cancer research, the National Cancer Institute (NCI) launched 12 physical science oncology centers at universities around the United States in 2009. The funders hoped that cancer research, which has benefited from tools made by physicists, also could benefit from physicists' unique perspective on cancer as a physical system.

Among the directors of the NCI centers, Princeton University's Robert Austin holds perhaps the most controversial perspective on cancer. Austin, a physicist and a member of the National Academy of Sciences, believes we might have cancer for a reason. It's a tradeoff that the rapid evolution our species has leveraged to become the dominant force on the planet. He suggested that cancer might act as a form of global population control, possibly serving to increase species fitness, in the following interview with Chris Palmer:[23]

> Q: What does all this say for whether we will ever find a cure for cancer?
> A: We should stop using the word "cure." It's the wrong word to use. We don't want to cure cancer. We have to have cancer to evolve. The hope is that you can keep cancer under control for a long enough time to die from something else.

Q: Should we just give up on chemotherapy?

A: No, no. I don't think we should give up on chemo, per se. We just do it in a simpleminded way right now. We give patients as much as they can tolerate. Instead of trying to kill the cancer, we should try to maintain it. In other words, maybe we should feed the tumor instead of starving it. Avastin was this anti-angiogenesis drug meant to starve a tumor by cutting off its blood supply. That drug has failed miserably. These cells simply evolved the ability to survive on less blood. They actually ended up more dangerous than if they hadn't given any drug at all. So, by starving them, we actually created an absolute monster.

Q: So, we should try to keep the tumor happy?

A: Yeah. Keep it happy and quiet. Can we learn to do that? I think that's not impossible.

A similar viewpoint is expressed by George Johnson in his book *The Cancer Chronicles*.[24] He says that as people age their cells amass more potentially cancerous mutations. Given a long enough life, cancer will eventually kill you—unless you die of something else first. He says that would be true even in a world free of carcinogens and equipped with the most powerful medical technology.

In his 2014 book *On The Cancer Frontier*, Dr. Paul Marks, former head of the Memorial Sloan-Kettering Cancer Center, says that the goal with cancer should be containment, not victory, because the enemy is uniquely intractable: "Medical science has never faced a more inscrutable, more mutable, or more ruthless adversary."[25]

Chemical and environmental polluting industries could well use these three viewpoints to discourage efforts to prevent cancer, as they do by debunking global warming.

Compromised Quality of Health Care in General

The questionable quality of health care generally received by patients in the United States compared to other economically developed nations needs to be recognized. Insurers, pharmaceutical companies and physicians have the largest financial stake in the system and have collectively presented barriers to finding real solutions for positive change.

Federal lawsuits charging Novartis Pharmaceuticals, the American subsidiary of a Swiss-based multinational, with making kickbacks to promote sales of its drugs raise disturbing questions about how to control fraudulent behavior in the pharmaceutical industry, behavior that appears to be on the rise, according to *The New York Times* Editorial Board.[26] Fines against other companies have not turned the tide against fraud. Stronger remedies are needed, perhaps including higher civil penalties for each fraudulent transaction and criminal prosecutions of the company officials responsible.

In today's global health industry, outright fraud, while real, does not pose the greatest threat to an individual's care. In his book *Bad Pharma: How Drug Companies Mislead Doctors and Harm Patients*, Dr. Ben Goldacre touches on the "ethical morass" of human trials and the "dirty tricks" pharmaceutical firms use to market their drugs both to patients and to doctors.[27] His book describes the poorly designed trials and outright testing manipulations that have led to "a market flooded with drugs that aren't very good." For years, researchers have talked about publication bias and selective publishing of positive rather than negative results of trials. Goldacre notes that only about half of clinical trials make their way into scientific journals.

The Downside of the Cancer Culture

As a psychiatrist, I am especially interested in what it is like for those who work in the cancer field. I suspect that one of the obvious, yet seldom conscious, reasons for adhering to conventional therapies is that oncology is the only medical field that depends upon the existence of a disease.

In my field, I run into unwitting resistance to working on preventing child abuse and neglect, the products of which create enormous expenditures and a lot of jobs. I try to reassure professionals who work with the products of child abuse and neglect that fluorides did not put dentists out of business, nor did vaccines health care workers. They still are reluctant to takes steps that would prevent the formation of dysfunctional families and strengthen struggling families. Their paradigm is based on providing interventions after problems arise in this way paralleling contemporary oncology.

Antibiotics and vaccines removed infectious diseases from prominence in medicine, but they did not threaten physicians because few depended upon these diseases for their livelihood. Although there were specialists in these diseases, they were basically pediatricians, internists, neurologists, etc.

The idea of a cure for cancer threatens the prominence, and perhaps the very existence, of the cancer field and its enormous number of facilities and expenditures. Actually, however, since cancer is a product of the biological process of neoplasia it really is not appropriate to imagine a cure for cancer. The best we can ever hope to do is prevent and control the process of neoplasia. Oncologists most likely always will be needed.

Conclusion

Understandably, professionals want to minimize the stress that arises when persons are informed that they have a life-threatening form of cancer. This leads them to put a positive face on their efforts to reassure and help patients and also to sustain their own sense of purpose and usefulness in their work. It also results in incomplete communication about cancer between professionals and patients and the public.

More important is the failure to act upon the obvious causes of cancer. The War on Cancer has focused far too much on treatment and not nearly enough on prevention. Political inaction to reduce environmental carcinogens is rooted in the influence of chemical companies—both those that profit by making pesticides and other cancer causing chemicals and those that profit by making cancer drugs. Preventing cancer means cleaning up our environment, green politics and dietary reform.

The "businessification" of medicine clearly distorts priorities in the cancer field. Over-diagnosis also is seen in the popular media promoting fear of cancer and perpetuating the myth that early aggressive treatment is always best; in the way doctors must take care to avoid lawsuits and in the profits made from screenings, medical procedures and pharmaceuticals.

Alternative medicine can be helpful, but it is an unregulated industry under no legal obligation to prove its claims or admit its risks and can actually be harmful to our health. Any therapy—alternative or traditional—should be scrutinized, and an agent that hasn't been shown to be safe and effective should not be called "medicine".

Recent questions raised about the reproducibility of biological and medical research findings are forcing scientists to embark on a soul-searching mission. Researchers are aware of publication bias and selective publishing of positive rather than negative results of trials.

The astounding view that we might have cancer as a form of global population control serving to increase species fitness and the view of cancer as an inevitable product of aging can be used to discourage cancer prevention.

The cancer culture need not fear winning the War on Cancer. The best we can ever hope for is preventing and controlling the bodily process of neoplasia. Oncologists always will be needed.

Chapter Fifteen

Where Do We Go from Here?

The ongoing impetus for change in the cancer field is described.

One of the basic tenets of clinical medicine is to do no harm. This presumes that the role of physicians is to aid the natural, life-sustaining forces of our bodies and minds in dealing with illnesses and injuries that impair our health. As examples, surgeons rely upon our bodies' capacities to heal, and primary care physicians rely upon our bodies' capacities to fend off infections after antibiotics have reduced the number of offending bacteria.

If we lose the capacity to heal naturally because our immune systems are overwhelmed, such as by drug-resistant viruses, bacteria, cancer or AIDS, we die. In other words, physicians do not cure any disease or fix any injury without relying upon our bodies' natural defenses. The "search for cancer and destroy it" model of oncology is not based on this fact and actually harms the body's natural defenses. This is the fundamental flaw in the conventional approach to cancer as if it is a disease in itself…get rid of cancer cells, and you cure cancer.

In order to think clearly about the way health care should work, the field of public health employs the concepts of primary, secondary and tertiary prevention. Primary prevention is preventing a disease or harm from occurring in the first place. Secondary prevention is treating a disease or harm. Tertiary prevention is minimizing the disability from a disease or harm.

In applying the public health approach to cancer, oncology employs primary prevention by identifying genetic and environmental factors that contribute to developing cancer, such as smoking, air pollution and toxic food contents (prevent neoplasia). Secondary prevention is employed in treatments that aim to cure cancer (stop neoplasia). Tertiary prevention is managing the course of cancer (slowing down neoplasia and palliative care).

Clinical oncologists are largely engaged in tertiary prevention because there is no cure for cancer as such. For example, the surgical removal of a tumor does not ensure that cancer will not recur. Chemotherapy aims to prolong survival from cancer. As an example, Vemurafenib was one of the first treatments for melanoma. It can cause tumors to shrivel within weeks. Unfortunately, continual mutation of the tumor creates resistant cancer cells, and most tumors rebound between six and nine months later.

Paradoxically, according to Meghna Das Thakur of the Novartis Institutes for Biomedical Research, in Emeryville, California, if cancer cells evolve with resistance to the chemotherapy being used to treat it, withdrawing that drug can sometimes stop the cancer in its tracks as effectively as the chemotherapy did in the first place.[1] This is because stopping the drug also stops suppressing the immune system, which then can destroy the newly mutated cancer cells that are unable to evade it as did the original cancer cells. In fact, this is the explanation for long-term remissions after chemotherapy...the immune system takes over and stops or restrains neoplasia. Believing that the chemotherapy drug did it all by itself is a dangerous fantasy.

Unfortunately, the many forms and the refractory nature of cancer have made it difficult to think clearly about principles to guide research that will have a significant impact. Fortunately, progress has been made in primary prevention that actually is the main reason for the decreases in cancer rates. Examples are smoking cessation programs that have reduced lung cancer and human papillomavirus vaccination that has reduced cervical cancer in women and oropharyngeal cancers in men. However, the knowledge that we have about how cancer cells develop and spread through neoplasia has not been given a high enough priority in secondary prevention clinical practice.

The Experience of Pediatric Oncology

Progress in the management of children with cancer has been hailed as one of the success stories of modern medicine. There has been a dramatic improvement in outcome for almost every category of childhood cancer. For childhood acute lymphoblastic leukemia (ALL)—the most common childhood cancer, which accounts for almost 30% of cases—the progress has been most gratifying. This is a disease that was virtually incurable in the 1960s. In the most recent trials, 5-year survival among children with ALL has approached 90%—truly significant progress over five decades.

What are the lessons that can be learned from the experience of pediatric oncology, and what are the implications for cancer care in general? First and foremost, caring for patients with cancer and restoring them to health require wide-ranging collaboration of diagnosticians, therapists and support services. It takes a village. Unfortunately, for most patients care remains fragmented and uncoordinated.

One of the reasons for its success has been that pediatric oncology pioneered the multidisciplinary approach to patients. There was early recognition of the need to collaborate beyond the confines of individual institutions. Among the most productive collaborations have been partnerships between clinicians and laboratory investigators, which allowed rapid incorporation of laboratory findings into the clinic.

What's more, Dr. Michael Link notes that a contributing factor may be based on what oncologist Dr. George Sledge calls "stupid" and "smart" cancers. Stupid cancers are responsive to treatment, whereas smart cancers evade therapy by developing resistance. The degree of stupidity can be quantified by the number of detectable mutations in a tumor. Compared with stupid cancers with few mutations, smart cancers, such as melanoma and lung cancer, have a more than 100-fold increase in the number of mutations. A majority of childhood cancers would qualify as stupid in Sledge's classification and are responsive to treatment.

Another factor is the maturing immune system in young people that makes it possible for an increasing capacity to prevent and stop neoplasia.

This raises the possibility that an encounter with cancer during early life may act as an immunization to that cancer in subsequent years.

Amid good news about progress in the management of childhood cancers, there are sobering reminders that we still have work to do. If we examine the mortality from childhood cancer as the rate plotted against year of diagnosis over time, the progress that has been made is clear. Also clear is that the curve has plateaued since 2000—and that further advancement is more difficult to demonstrate. It is evident that we have squeezed what we can from conventional chemotherapeutic agents.

Link calls for a new paradigm—one that will involve yet further collaboration if we are to make greater progress.[2] The genomic era has brought stunning advances in our understanding of the biology of cancer. Understanding tumors on a biologic basis is necessary to determine the most appropriate therapy. If childhood ALL has taught us anything, Link said it is that we should be astonished that our crude, empirical therapies have been successful at all, especially in light of today's understanding that we have been treating an assortment of diseases with distinct genetic profiles having little relation to each other.

Link added that these lessons from our children emphasize the challenges that face us in caring for adults with cancer. We do not yet understand which molecular pathways are most important; our current clinical trial designs are inadequate for the era of personalized medicine and we are just beginning to realize the potential of health information technology. To address these challenges, ASCO's 2011 report *Accelerating Progress Against Cancer* includes a discussion of new approaches to cancer drug development, to trial designs with participants selected on the basis of the molecular features of their tumors and to what can be harnessed from health information technology.

In the management of cancer, our best strategy would move us from the paradigm of "diagnose and treat" to one of "predict and prevent". Here, too, pediatricians may hold the key—because the best opportunity to prevent cancers in adults is proper immunization and lifestyle counseling of children. Successful immunization against hepatitis B and human papillomavirus (at ages 11 or 12) presents the prospect of preventing much of hepatocellular carcinoma and cervical cancer and perhaps a substantial portion of oropharyngeal cancers as well. We can only hope for equally successful vaccines against Epstein-Barr virus, hepatitis C and Helicobacter pylori. Pediatricians also can influence children and families to promote healthy lifestyles and to educate them about the dangers of smoking, obesity and ultraviolet exposure—the major risk factors for preventable adult cancers.

Link concluded: "What really underlies the success of pediatric oncology? It's the culture of collaboration and learning that permeates our specialty. It's the seamless integration of clinical research with medical practice, the collection of tissues for study as a key component of research and a remarkable level of participation by physicians and patients in the clinical research process. It's the understanding by physicians, patients and their families that clinical research is the key vehicle for progress."

The National Cancer Institute is Moving Forward

The NCI Budget Proposal for 2012 noted that advances accrued over the past decade of cancer research have fundamentally changed the conversations that Americans can have about cancer.[3] The 2012 Proposal said that, although many still think of cancer as a single disease affecting different parts of the body, research tells us—through new tools and technologies, massive computing power and new insights from other fields—cancer is, in fact, a collection of many diseases whose ultimate number, causes and treatment represent a challenging biomedical puzzle. Unfortunately, this view is not very encouraging and does not mention neoplasia as a fundamental biological process in the body.

At the same time, the NCI Budget Proposal went on to say:

> We now know that cancer is caused by changes in a cell's genetic makeup and its programmed behavior. Sometimes these changes are spontaneous, and sometimes they arise from environmental or behavioral triggers, such as ultraviolet radiation from sunlight or

chemicals in tobacco smoke. We have at hand the methods to identify essentially all of the genomic changes in a cell and to use that knowledge to rework the landscape of cancer research, from basic science to prevention, diagnosis, and treatment.

This knowledge brings us—and our national conversation—to a crucial opportunity for acceleration in the study of cancer and its treatment. The emerging scientific landscape offers the promise of significant advances for current and future cancer patients, just as it offers scientists at the National Cancer Institute—and in the thousands of laboratories across the United States that receive NCI support—the opportunity to dramatically increase the pace of lifesaving discoveries where progress has long been steady but mostly incremental.

The Budget Proposal does speak positively about the possibility of identifying the bodily processes that underlie the development of cancer cells (neoplasia).

We have identified proteins and pathways that different cancers may have in common and represent targets for new drugs for these and many other cancers—since so often research in one cancer creates potential benefits across others.

The Budget Proposal concludes that:

We reap the rewards of investments in cancer made over the past 40 years or more, even as we stake out a bold investment strategy to realize the potential we see so clearly. No matter what the fiscal climate, NCI will strive to commit the resources necessary to bring about a new era of cancer research, diagnosis, prevention, and treatment. A fair share of those resources will be committed to the technical work required to understand the full dimensions of the molecular basis of cancer, coupled with the intricate analyses that translate that understanding into actionable strategies to reduce the burden of cancer. Cancer research, perhaps more than the study of any malady, involves the deepest knowledge of human biology.

It's understandable that NCI would desire to present a positive view about the progress that has been made in the cancer field if it is to be a credible recipient of federal funds. This is especially understandable when the funding history of NCI, reviewed earlier in Chapter Thirteen, is examined.

Movements Devoted to Improving Cancer Care

Cancer research—indeed, most medical research—is typically about the narrowly focused investigator with one small grant at a time. But advances in genetic profiling of cancers and the mutations that cause them are telling scientists and physicians they must stop working in silos and stop treating lung or breast or colon or prostate cancer as distinct diseases. Common genetic mutations, like one called p53 that controls cell death, are showing up across a whole swath of cancers. A mutation called BRCA1 is common in women's cancers, such as breast and ovarian, yet the research and clinical work in those two diseases has largely been separate.

My personal explorations and conclusions derived from published NCI data and discussions with NCI staff members confirm the American Association of Clinical Oncology's 2011 assertion that cancer research and care must be vastly improved. A number of organizations are taking advantage of this opportunity to move toward a sea change in the cancer field. Among the most prominent are the following.

Nation Academy of Sciences

As mentioned in Chapter Two, the need for change in the cancer field was affirmed at a National Academy of Sciences Workshop in 2013 devoted to improving the affordability and quality of cancer care.[4] A recurring theme of the workshop was the need for all stakeholders—including patients, clinicians, private and government payers and the pharmaceutical and device industries—to work together to address improving cancer care. Because cancer is such a prevalent set of conditions and so costly, it exposes all of the strengths and weaknesses of our health care system in general. The workshop suggested that oncology is where the action for change is going to be in health care.

Stand Up to Cancer (SU2C)

In his 2013 *Time* magazine article on cancer, Bill Saporito quoted the Massachusetts Institute of Technology's Philip Sharp: "This disease is much more complex than we have been treating it. And the complexity is stunning."[5] Sharp—a Nobel Prize-winning molecular biologist who studies the genetic causes of cancer—is recruiting special-forces units to fight cancer. For the past four years, he has been wrangling "dream teams" funded by SU2C, an organization started by entertainment-industry celebrities unhappy with the progress being made against cancer.

What does it take to transform the way an entire medical ecosystem functions, Saporito asks? In this case, an unprecedented combination of celebrities, intensity and large amounts of money. In 2008 a group including Spider-Man producer Laura Ziskin, who lost her battle with breast cancer in 2011; Katie Couric, who lost her husband to colon cancer in 1998 and former Paramount CEO Sherry Lansing founded SU2C with the goal of attacking cancer the way you make a movie: bring the best and most talented possible people together, fund them generously, oversee their progress rigorously and shoot for big payoffs—on a tight schedule.

SU2C raises money through foundations in addition to corporate, organizational and private donors and then grants it to teams in the form of unusually large sums (up to $18 million, vs. about $500,000 for a typical grant from the National Institutes of Health) to produce results in a short time, initially three years. All the chosen projects are monitored by the American Association for Cancer Research. A SU2C scientific committee headed by Philip Sharp and other heavy hitters reviews each team semiannually, a checkup that can make top scientists feel like graduate students. "When you have to answer to Nobel laureates and others, it's a very tough review team," Dr. Daniel Von Hoff, physician in chief at the Translational Genomics Research Institute—a dream team launched by SU2C that's studying pancreatic cancer, said to Saporito.

The team model also is disrupting the normal course of business across the medical-research community. For investigators, it means changes in the way careers are developed, the way data are shared and especially the way credit for achievement is shared. For institutions, team research means changes in contracts, compensation, titles and the own-ership of intellectual property. For pharmaceutical companies, it means restructuring the way experimental drugs are allocated and clinical trials are conducted.

NCI, which has parceled out its $5.5 billion cancer-research budget to a single principal investigator for each grant it makes, is recognizing the paradigm shift in its PPG and SPORES programs. National Institute of Health Director Dr. Francis Collins, who led the team at the Human Genome Project, said that under his watch, the 27 institutes he oversees will be less independent fiefdoms pursuing their own goals and more trustworthy collaborators that can team up to answer common and com-plex biomedical questions. "I am strongly anti-silo, strongly pro-break-ing-down-barriers, bringing disciplines together, building collaborations and building dream teams," he said.

Interdisciplinary Centers

An example of the growing interdisciplinary trend is the newly es-tablished cancer center at Weill Cornell Medical College and New York-Presbyterian Hospital on the Upper East Side of Manhattan that will bring together researchers in various fields—basic scientists, pathologists, surgeons, radiologists and more.[6] A joint effort with Memorial Sloan-Kettering Cancer Center, the Rockefeller University, and the Takeda Pharmaceutical Company, the institute will facilitate translation of early-stage drug discoveries into treatments. Dr. Lewis C. Cantley, director of the Center said, "In the past, even with chemotherapy and radiation, we didn't know why some people responded and some didn't; now with these targeted therapies, we do know. It's not, 'Let's randomly try another set of poisons and see what happens.' Because that's what we've been doing for thirty years."

One Small Victory at a Time

Saporito gives a case example of how the treatment of cancer is changing.[7] As if the lung cancer that had defied conventional therapies had not been enough, the metastatic tumors in and around Tom Stanback's lungs grew so large that he was having difficulty swallowing and breathing. Unwilling to go quietly, Stanback actively sought out clinical trials in search of anything that might extend his life. One of them, at Johns Hopkins in Baltimore, is focused on studying the enzymatic on/off switches that sit atop the underlying genes and regulate whether and how loudly those genes will be expressed. This includes the mutated genes that crank out cancer cells. While science can't do much to change the genes, epigenetic functions are manipulated all of the time—sometimes inadvertently by exposure to environmental chemicals other times cleverly by drugs. Stanback, a 62-year-old, 40-year former smoker, was involved in a trial to see if a new epigenetic drug could shrink his tumors.

In Stanback's case, the answer was no, not quite. But the leaders of the cross-disciplinary, cross-institutional research team behind the work (one of 10 dream teams backed by SU2C) weren't finished. They postulated that even if the epigenetic manipulation alone didn't knock out the cancer, it could have a priming effect, improving the likelihood that other treatments administered later would work. That's exactly what happened when Stanback returned home for a round of radiation therapy at Memorial Sloan-Kettering Cancer Center in New York City and joined a second clinical trial. His tumors shrank markedly in the past year and a half and were not visible on a subsequent CT scan. "The drug nudges the T cells to being alive and active," he said. "I'm alive. I'm healthier than I've ever been." Even better, other patients in the study have enjoyed what appear to be complete remissions.

The team behind these accomplishments is led by Dr. Stephen Baylin, an oncologist at Johns Hopkins, and Dr. Peter Jones, a biochemist and molecular biologist at the University of Southern California. They ride herd on a diverse group of experts—geneticists, pathologists, biostatisticians, biochemists, oncologists, surgeons, nurses, technicians and specialists who normally wouldn't have been working as an ensemble. The team was awarded its grant in May 2009 and within the year was able to extend the epigenetic clinical trial that enrolled Stanback and launch new ones. That is light speed in modern research—the lab to clinic cycle in cancer is typically a decade.

Saporito noted that this kind of institutional transformation is not easy, but it's the only way to take advantage of the dazzling scientific and technological advances that have taken place in just the past three years. Sequencing the first human genome took more than a decade and $2.7 billion. Today sequencing can be done for a few thousand dollars in a few hours.

That progress has led to similar pharmaceutical leaps. Hundreds of drugs are in development for therapies targeting neoplasia. Some, as in the case of Stanback's trial, seek to reactivate the body's immune system. Others are designed to cut off a tumor's blood or energy supply; still others seek to restart apoptosis, the programmed cell death that normally takes place in healthy bodies. New biomarkers are allowing doctors to identify, target and track cancer cells. "It happened, and it happened quickly," said DePinho. "If you look back on the progress that we made, it was against not having a periodic table of cancer, of not being able to understand genes, of not being able to model."

Today the physics of cancer are known; what remains is massive engineering. "In the old days, everyone knew it took 30 years to test a compound," said Dr. Daniel Haber, director of the Massachusetts General Hospital Cancer Center. Scientists got that to an eight-to-10-year process. Teams of researchers are trying to whittle it down to a two-year timeline. That's fast by most measures—but not fast enough if you're a patient. Said Haber: "Cancer doesn't wait two years."

Saporito wisely cautions that despite that urgency, shifting to a team model will not be easy, in part because "the sociology of medical research isn't very social." Historically, the principal investigator wins grant money for a proposal and takes top billing on everything from publications to patents to the glory that goes with them. Those outcomes in turn are crucial to getting more grants. It's self-perpetuating and self-limiting and over the past decade has increasingly stifled young investigators in particular because the percentage of grant applications that are funded by NIH, the so-called pay line, is now below 10% and falling.

Team science demands that top researchers work with other top researchers and share an investigation, the data and the credit. Baylin and Jones, leaders of SU2C's epigenetics team, were rivals for years. "It does take an ego to do this business," said Baylin, "because everybody is more than ready to tell you you're wrong." For these two, things have warmed up so much that their families have vacationed together.

Haber, an oncologist, has similarly partnered with Massachusetts General biomedical engineer Mehmet Toner to lead an SU2C-backed team that has designed and built a smart chip device to trap circulating tumor cells (CTCs) in a blood sample. Many tumors release cells into the bloodstream; if a CTC settles in another organ and starts to grow, that's metastasis. The breakaway cells are not easy to spot—there are a billion blood cells for every one of them—but detecting their presence is critical to stopping their spread.

The business-card-size detector the team built uses antibodies that bind to certain cell proteins to isolate and capture the CTCs. It's possible the device will change the standard of care for treating several cancers, beginning with metastatic prostate cancer. The CTC chip's role as a hunter-trapper is also being applied to lung cancer, where mutations can help direct powerful new therapies, to see how CTCs change and evolve during the course of treatment. With other cancers, like pancreatic cancer, where there are currently no mutations that can be targeted, CTCs are being analyzed to see if they can reveal new vulnerabilities in tumor cells.

Saporito concluded that lassoing a single blood cell is complicated enough. But pairing bioengineers with oncologists is no small thing either, at least until they are brought together by an NCI or SU2C grant. "The field had a bad rep and wasn't moving forward," said Haber, "but they learned DNA, and we learned equations." His team even includes an entrepreneur-in-residence, Dr. Ravi Kapur, who was in charge of rolling out the prototype to the team's collaborating institutions.

Big Pharma, Big Results

Saporito aptly describes cancer as a thief and biological con artist, breaking into and taking control of the mechanisms of a cell and coaxing it to grow and divide in dangerous ways. Dr. Lewis Cantley has spent a career chasing this cellular saboteur by, as he described it, "teasing out signaling pathways" that govern not just growth but the very life span of a cell. If the neoplastic signaling can be silenced or reversed, the cancer cells won't spread. In pursuit of that goal, he is now a co-leader of a team backed by SU2C that targets a pathway called PI3K. The pathway is a known driver in three women's cancers: ovarian, endometrial and especially breast, which involves the PI3K mutation in 30% of cases. Said Cantley: "It's the most frequently mutated oncogene in cancer."

Drug companies have long been targeting mutations like this one to develop compounds that will interfere with the defective biochemical gateways. There are hundreds of drugs that may have some effect against some of the mutations, which sounds like an abundance of riches—but it's also an abundance of complexity. That's one reason that the pharma industry has a 95% failure rate for new products and that half of Phase III trials—the last step before approval—don't cut it. "If I have 100 different drugs I can use in combination, then 100 times 100 is 10,000. You can't do 10,000 trials," said MIT's Philip Sharp.

But which ones can you do and should you do and on which patients?

Since PI3K mutations are the most common type, those seemed like a perfect place to start for Cantley's dream team, which is co-led by Dr. Gordon Mills of MD Anderson—another world-class PI3K pathway investigator—along with women's-cancer specialists from Massachusetts General Hospital, Vanderbilt University, Columbia University, Beth Israel Deaconess Hospital and Memorial Sloan-Kettering. The team needed a PI3K inhibitor from Novartis and a PARP inhibitor from AstraZeneca. Neither drug is approved for cancer treatment, and it's rare to conduct a trial in which two unapproved drugs are combined. Because of concerns about intellectual property and other issues—no drugmaker wants to be smeared by the toxicity of another's drug—companies are wary of collaboration.

Still, the success of the Cantley-Mills team had drug firms lining up. "Every company that had a PI3K inhibitor called me and asked would I work with them," said Cantley. The result was almost without precedent: a human trial at five institutions with two unapproved drugs from two companies within about a year of discovery. "Four years ago if you said you were going to do that, you would have been laughed out of the room." The goal now is to launch trials as rapidly as the geneticists and biochemists solve the equation of matching mutations with drug compounds.

Moon Shots program

Saporito described the Moon Shots program. Dr. Ronald DePinho, president of MD Anderson Cancer Center, adopted a collaborative approach around what the Center calls its Moon Shots program, assembling six multidisciplinary groups to mount comprehensive attacks on eight cancers: lung, prostate, melanoma, breast, ovarian and three types of leukemia. For DePinho, this is a $3 billion throwdown. He's backing his teams massively, with plans for $300 million annually over the next decade by reallocating existing research funds and soliciting new donations. As in the SU2C effort, teams will be judged by patient outcomes, not by the number of research papers published. "Aspiring is not enough. You must achieve," he says. "It's about integration across the entire cancer continuum, and it's about execution. People will be judged by whether they have reduced mortality in cancer."

DePinho's use of the moon-shot analogy goes back to 1961, when President John F. Kennedy announced that the U.S. was going to the moon, and the idea was no longer science fiction. The physics were understood. What remained was a giant engineering project. Apply enough money and aerospace engineers and you eventually get to Neil Armstrong's giant leap for mankind. When President Richard Nixon announced the War on Cancer in 1971, victory wasn't even as remotely possible as going to the moon had been in 1961. There were no physics to build upon. It was as if someone had announced a moon shot for cancer in 1820.

"Exploiting connections," Dr. John Heymach, an oncologist at MD Anderson and member of a SU2C dream team, told Saporito "is where team science becomes important. It's a pattern-recognition exercise. We are going to accumulate data and expertise. We are going to profile all these different mutations."

Bree Sandlin is among the thousands of patients at MD Anderson rooting for the Moon Shots program. She's a 37-year-old marketing executive for Shell who has twin boys and triple-negative breast cancer—so named because receptors for estrogen, progesterone and a growth factor known as HER-2/neu are missing. This makes treatment difficult, since those are targets for hormone and drug therapies. She's in a clinical trial that is testing the effectiveness of eribulin, a cancer drug typically used in metastatic breast cancer, as an immune system kick-starter. So far, it's working well. "That approach to research is just very different than how they used to approach it in the past," she says. "It can't help but give me hope."

More hope for other potential patients is coming from the primary prevention focus on prevention and early detection. If patients like Sandlin are genetically predisposed to breast cancer, what about other women in the family? If they are offered testing for the same biomarkers, the doctors could head off big trouble by catching any cancer early.

Likewise, there are 94 million ex-smokers in the U.S. with elevated cancer risks. Subjecting each of them to an annual CT scan would catch early-stage lung cancers and reduce mortality from the disease by perhaps

20%. Given that there are 175,000 new lung cancers diagnosed every year, that's a lot of lives. But getting all those people into a CT machine is neither practical nor even possible. Instead, MD Anderson and other cancer centers are developing simple blood tests that could, when used in combination with diagnostic imaging and risk models, detect lung cancer earlier than it is typically found.

"It's a measure, perhaps, of what a quagmire the War on Cancer has become that the basic premise of the whole enterprise—that this is about saving lives—requires repeating," concluded Saporito.

The Long Shot: Pancreatic Cancer

For all the progress made against some types of cancer, there are others that have never been anything but bad news. Take pancreatic cancer, an area that Philip Sharp bluntly labeled "a disaster" for Saporito. The cancer often is discovered in a late stage, and most tumors are inoperable. They're smart cancer cells that resist treatment. The goal of Daniel Von Hoff of the Translational Genomics Research Institute in Phoenix, Arizona, who leads SU2C's pancreatic dream team along with Craig Thompson, CEO of Memorial Sloan-Kettering, is to improve survival rates. Currently, less than 25% of patients with advanced pancreatic cancer make it to one year.

The focus of the 28-person team scattered across five institutions is to better understand the metabolic changes that characterize pancreatic cells. It's a collaborative exercise that starts when surgeon Jeffrey Drebin of the University of Pennsylvania removes a tumor from a diseased pancreas. He carries it from the operating room to a lab, where it is flash-frozen for preservation. Penn's lab sends a specimen to the Salk Institute's Gene Expression Laboratory, where researcher Geoffrey Wahl and colleagues analyze the state of stellate, or star-shaped, cells that are usually involved in tissue repair but may play a role in cancer as well. Another sample goes to Princeton to the lab of Joshua Rabinowitz, who analyzes amino acids, sugar and up to 300 metabolites. Team members at Johns Hopkins and Translational Genomics analyze the genetic sequence.

One of the team's emerging theories is that pancreatic cancer cells communicate with stellate cells that also show up around the tumor and conspire to ward off immune responses and build resistance to chemotherapies. The tumor cells seem to leech glutamine and other amino acids from the rest of the body to feed the tumor—one reason people with pancreatic cancer lose so much weight. Prevent the hijacking of glutamine and other amino acids and perhaps the tumor will starve. The team also has discovered that vitamin D3 can help stop the scarring around the cancer and give the immune system or chemotherapies better access to cancer cells.

Team science isn't appropriate for every aspect of cancer research. Nor is it issue-free. Saporito found one question up for grabs: How long should a team be together? SU2C's initial funding is for three years, although some teams have secured money for additional years. The pancreatic team, for instance, received two grants of $2 million each from the Lustgarten Foundation and SU2C for another two years of work. At MD Anderson, DePinho is committed to the team concept, but he's also willing to defund or change the leadership of teams that don't perform. The state of Texas, following the team model, passed a $3 billion bond issue to fund cancer research, but the program apparently has been plagued by allegations of political intrigue and mismanagement.

Saporito believes that the traditional researcher, sitting alone or with a couple of postdocs in a lab somewhere, working on that eureka moment, will always have a niche in this new ecosystem. "We still need people looking under rocks," said Dr. William Nelson, director of the Johns Hopkins Cancer Center, a vice chairman of SU2C's scientific-advisory committee and a successful "rock looker underer", having discovered the most common genome alteration in prostate cancer. But the shift to team science is permanent. When he first considered SU2C's team structure, Drebin was skeptical. "My feeling was that this was naiveté on the part of Hollywood executives," he said. "You can make a movie this way. But not science. I take that back."

Preventing Neoplasia

Thus far we have been focusing on secondary and tertiary prevention. Just as important is the primary prevention of neoplasia.

There are a number of environmental factors that we know stimulate neoplasia. Foremost among them are ultraviolet light, smoking, asbestos, obesity, nuclear radiation, chemical and particulate air and water pollution and medical imaging radiation.

Ultraviolet light

Skin cancer is the most common form of cancer. The two most common types of skin cancer—basal cell and squamous cell carcinomas—can be removed by surgical procedures. However, melanoma, the third most common skin cancer, is more dangerous. The vast majority of melanomas are caused by exposure to ultraviolet light (UV) that is an invisible kind of radiation that comes from the sun, tanning beds and sunlamps. UV rays can penetrate and alter the DNA of skin cells.

The National Weather Service and the Environmental Protection Agency developed the UV Index to forecast the risk of overexposure to UV rays. It lets you know how much caution you should take when working, playing or exercising outdoors. The UV Index predicts exposure levels on a 1–15 scale with higher levels indicating a higher risk of overexposure. Calculated on a next-day basis for dozens of cities across the United States, the UV Index takes into account clouds and other local conditions that affect the amount of UV rays reaching the ground.

Smoking

Tobacco use is the leading cause of preventable illness and death in the United States. It causes different cancers as well as chronic lung and heart diseases.[8]

+ Cigarette smoking causes an estimated 443,000 deaths each year, including approximately 49,000 deaths due to exposure to secondhand smoke.
+ Lung cancer is the leading cause of cancer death among both men and women in the United States, and 90 percent of lung cancer

deaths among men and approximately 80 percent of lung cancer deaths among women are due to smoking.

- Smoking causes many other types of cancer, including cancers of the throat, mouth, nasal cavity, esophagus, stomach, pancreas, kidney, bladder and cervix in addition to acute myeloid leukemia.
- People who smoke are up to six times more likely to suffer a heart attack than nonsmokers, and the risk increases with the number of cigarettes smoked. Smoking also causes most cases of chronic lung disease.
- According to the Centers for Disease Control and Prevention, in 2012 an estimated 19 percent of U.S. adults were cigarette smokers; 23 percent of high school students used tobacco products.

Obesity

The American Cancer Society estimates that 1 out of every 3 cancer deaths in the United States is linked to excess body weight, poor nutrition and/or physical inactivity.[9] These factors are related and contribute to cancer risk, but excess body weight has the strongest evidence linking it to cancer and contributes to as many as 1 out of 5 of all cancer-related deaths. The percentage of cases attributed to obesity vary widely for different cancer types but is as high as 40 percent for some, particularly endometrial cancer and esophageal adenocarcinoma. One study projected that continuation of existing trends in obesity will lead to about 500,000 additional cases of cancer in the United States by 2030.

Several mechanisms have been suggested to explain the association of obesity with increased risk of certain cancers:[10]

- Obese people often have increased levels of insulin and insulin-like growth factor-1 (IGF-1) in their blood (a condition known as hyperinsulinemia or insulin resistance), which may promote the development of certain tumors.
- Fat cells produce a hormone, leptin, which seems to promote cell proliferation.

+ Fat cells also may have direct and indirect effects on other tumor growth regulators, including rapamycin (mTOR) and AMP-activated protein kinase.

+ Obese people often have chronic low-level, or "subacute", inflammation, which has been associated with increased cancer risk.

+ Fat tissue produces excess amounts of estrogen, high levels of which have been associated with the risk of breast, endometrial and some other cancers. Low density cholesterol that contributes to heart attacks and strokes has another nasty trick up its sleeve. When metabolized by the body, it turns into a potent estrogen-like molecule that spurs the growth of breast cancer in mice and perhaps in people.[11]

+ Other possible mechanisms include altered immune responses, effects on the nuclear factor kappa beta system and oxidative stress (free radicals).

Nuclear Radiation

As might be expected because of the financial considerations involved in energy produced from nuclear sources, the collection and interpretation of data on the impact of nuclear radiation on health and specifically on cancer has led to either minimizing or highlighting its long-term effects.

Among the long-term effects suffered by atomic bomb survivors in Hiroshima and Nagasaki, the most deadly was leukemia. The Radiation Effects Research Foundation, a Japan/U.S. organization, estimated the risk of leukemia to have been 46% for bomb victims peaking around four to six years later and most seriously affecting children.[12] For all other cancers, an incidence increase did not appear until around ten years after the attacks when the cancer risk was up to five times greater than the risk of an unexposed individual. Fetal exposure in utero also produced birth defects.

2013 marked the 25th anniversary of the Chernobyl nuclear plant accident. It came as nuclear industry and pro-nuclear government officials in the United States and other nations were trying to "revive" nuclear power. The World Health Organization's (WHO) 20-year review of the

Chernobyl disaster found that its psychological impacts did more health damage than radiation exposure, and a principle cause of the population's debilitating stress was "an exaggerated sense of the dangers to health of exposure to radiation."

In contrast with the WHO review, the controversial 2009 book from the Center for Russian Environmental Policy *Chernobyl: Consequences of the Catastrophe for People and the Environment* claimed to be the most comprehensive study ever made on the impacts of the Chernobyl disaster. It concluded that based on records available then, some 985,000 people died mainly of cancer between when the Chernobyl accident occurred in 1986 and 2004.[13] More deaths, it projected, will follow. The book claims that the International Atomic Energy Agency expected death toll from the Chernobyl accident of 4,000 extremely underestimates the casualties of Chernobyl. Although published by the *Annals of the New York Academy of Sciences*, this book was not peer reviewed.

Epidemiologists are studying Fukushima, Japan, where radiation exposures were far lower than at Chernobyl and are finding adverse psychological effects. The World Health Organization predicts minor increases in rates of some cancers for some ages and genders in small pockets of more highly contaminated areas near the plant. Nonetheless, thousands of people in the Fukushima disaster area refused to return to their homes and businesses in evacuated areas, even where dose levels had fallen low enough to declare those areas safe. Levels of stress, anxiety and depression are significantly elevated. One survey found that stress among children in the Fukushima area is double the level of other children in Japan. The Japanese Education Ministry reported that the children in Fukushima Prefecture have become the most obese in Japan since the nuclear accident prompted schools to curtail outside exercise, in most cases in areas where the risk from radiation was infinitesimal.

Environmental Pollution

The connection of cancer to toxic environmental pollutants has been made. It has long been known that smoking and secondary exposure to smoke is a precursor of lung cancer. Mesothelioma is a form of lung cancer sufficiently connected to asbestos exposure that compensation is available if that connection can be made.[14]

Growing interest is being shown in the influence of environmental toxins on genes and how that might lead normal cells to become cancer cells. This was brought home to Nancy and me by the deaths from breast cancer of two of our friends who lived next door to us in a new development, Kensington Farms, in Ann Arbor, Michigan. Our third neighbor died prematurely with multiple sclerosis. Three of our close neighbors had died prematurely years ago. We wondered if this could have been related to the development having been built on drainage from a waste dump.

The International Agency for Research on Cancer (IARC) identified 464 natural and artificial agents as having some level of carcinogenicity in humans.[15] With some overlap, a catalogue by the U. S. National Toxicology Program (USNTP) lists 240 substances as "known" or "reasonably anticipated" human carcinogens. Some cancer-causing agents occur naturally, such as poisonous compounds produced by molds that grow in nuts, seeds and legumes. Others are human-made, such as ionizing radiation from medical imaging and various commercial chemicals. Yet of the 80,000 chemicals in our environment, only a tiny fraction has been tested for carcinogenicity.

Designating a substance as a carcinogen and making recommendations about its use can be controversial. For example, in 2011, the USNTP listed formaldehyde, a chemical commonly used in building materials and household products, as a carcinogen, and styrene, which is used to make plastics and rubber, as reasonably anticipated to be a human carcinogen. Despite similar designations by the IARC and other agencies, industry groups such as the American Chemistry Council successfully advocated for a review of the report by the National Academies in an effort to get the chemicals delisted and avoid further regulation.

Three compelling themes have emerged from studies of environmental factors in breast cancer. First, breast cancer is now recognized as a developmental disease with windows of susceptibility across the life course, beginning in the womb, during puberty and the early reproductive years and up to the 5 years before diagnosis. Second, laboratory studies in rodents reveal hundreds of common chemicals that activate biological pathways, including chemicals that cause mammary gland tumors, hormone disruptors that interact with the estrogen receptor and promote tumor proliferation and developmental toxicants that alter mammary gland development in ways that later affect lactation and cancer susceptibility. Third, the U.S. National Report on Human Exposure to Environmental Chemicals and other exposure studies show that these suspect chemicals are widespread in air and water pollution, consumer products, house dust and human tissues.[16]

As with nuclear radiation, air pollution and global warming, direct chemical pollution of water and soil is subject to minimization by commercial interests. The Love Canal scandal in upstate New York was based upon an increase in health problems, especially birth defects, but it was reported to have resulted in only a slight increase in cancer by the New York Department of Health.[17]

Marines and Navy personnel stationed at Camp Lejeune in North Carolina between 1975 and 1985 when its drinking water was highly polluted with toxic chemicals died of cancer far more frequently than those who lived at a base without fouled water.[18]

Over the past decade, Erin Brockovich has received hundreds of thousands of emails from people around the United States and the globe reporting problems that they were experiencing in their communities.[19] Many of these inquiries were about environmental concerns. She acts as the voice of the people who on a daily basis are experiencing the harmful effects of water, air and soil pollution in their communities. She created a map to help better understand what might really be going on.

The Centers for Disease Control and Prevention (CDCP) states that confirmation of a cancer cluster does not necessarily mean that there is any single, external cause or hazard that can be addressed. A confirmed cancer cluster could be the result of any of the following:

+ chance
+ miscalculation of the expected number of cancer cases (e.g., not considering a risk factor within the population at risk)

+ differences in the case definition between observed cases and expected cases
+ known causes of cancer (e.g., smoking)
+ unknown cause(s) of cancer

The CDCP compiles a list of reported clusters recorded according to specific standards and notes that follow-up investigations can take years to complete with generally inconclusive results.[20]

Polyvinyl Chloride

Scientists in Virginia reported in 2008 that home plumbing systems constructed with polyvinyl chloride (PVC) plastic pipes may be more susceptible to leaching of lead and copper into drinking water than other types of piping—especially when PVC systems include brass fixtures and pipe fittings.[21]

Previous studies found that ammonia formed in chloramine-treated water (instead of chlorination) can trigger a series of events that corrode brass faucet components and connectors commonly used in PVC plumbing systems. Corrosion of brass (made with copper, zinc and lead) releases those metals into water pipes and makes faucets prone to failure.

In another study, researchers sampled water from PVC, copper, lead and other pipe material under a range of experimental conditions.[22] They found that corrosive conditions were often worst in plastic pipes, which could be expected to cause higher metal leaching of zinc and lead from brass faucets used in homes and buildings.

PVC can be manufactured as flexible or rigid. Flexible PVC is used for medical bags, shower curtains, shrink wrap and deli and meat wrap. Rigid PVC comprises 70% of all manufactured PVC. It is used to make construction materials such as pipe, siding, window frames, railing, fencing and decking. PVC has made a major contribution to improving the conveniences of life around the world.

In addition to the toxic pollution PVC itself creates, it also commonly has toxic additives, so it's impacting your health just through everyday use.

According to the Center for Health, Environment, and Justice (CHEJ), the production of PVC requires chemicals like the "cancer-causing" vinyl chloride monomer and ethylene dichloride. The CHEJ points out that PVC plastic requires large amounts of toxic additives to make it stable and usable.[23] These additives are released during use and disposal, resulting in "elevated human exposures to phthalates, lead, cadmium, tin and other toxic chemicals."

Workers in PVC manufacturing facilities and residents of surrounding communities are at risk from exposure to these chemicals which contaminate the water, soil and air around these facilities. On February 13, 2012, the Environmental Protection Agency issued a rule that requires facilities producing PVC to reduce emissions of harmful toxic air emissions to protect public health in communities where these facilities are located.

The Food and Drug Administration acknowledged that the building block of PVC, vinyl chloride, is a human carcinogen. It concluded that the amount contained in PVC food packaging is within safe limits. In 2002, the FDA recommended that a specific compound used as a plasticizer in PVC either be labeled or removed from the medical bags in which it was being used. This compound, DEHP, has shown toxic and carcinogenic effects in lab animals. The body-invasive medical procedures in which these bags are being used may expose people to DEHP levels that exceed the amount determined to be safe in humans.

A study by researchers from Cornell University, Stanford University, and the Virginia Polytechnic Institute found cancer-causing vinyl chloride in water carried by PVC pipes.[24] The vinyl industry's view is that the vinyl chloride is bound to the plastic and doesn't leach. However, these scientists found that PVC/CPVC pipe reactors in the laboratory and water tap samples collected from homes revealed vinyl chloride accumulation in the tens of $\mu g/L$ range after a few days and hundreds of $\mu g/L$ after two years. While these levels did not exceed the EPA's maximum daily contaminant level of 2 $\mu g/L$, many readings that simulated stagnation times in homes overnight did. The most effective way to remove vinyl chloride in homes with PVC piping is through reverse osmosis water purification systems.

Some European Union (EU) nations already prohibit lead content in PVC pipes, widely used in urban water and wastewater systems and in home plumbing. The EU's main manufacturers of PVC pipes have voluntarily agreed to eliminate the use of lead as a stabilizer in the manufacturing process by 2015, following through on pledges first made in 2000.[25]

From both an environmental and health standpoint, PVC is the most toxic plastic. Here's why: vinyl chloride, the chemical used to make PVC, is a known human carcinogen, according to the World Health Organization's International Agency for Research on Cancer. The manufacture and incineration of PVC also creates and releases dioxins, which cause a wide range of health effects including cancer, birth defects, diabetes, learning and developmental delays, endometriosis and immune system abnormalities. One type of dioxin is the most potent carcinogen ever tested. It's nasty stuff.

Because dioxins are highly poisonous to the cells of our bodies, don't freeze plastic bottles with water in them or heat your food in the microwave using plastic containers or wraps as this releases dioxins from the plastic. Cover food with a paper towel and use glass, such as Corning Ware, Pyrex or ceramic containers, for heating such things as TV dinners and instant soups.

What happens to those environmental dioxins once they're released? They end up in the food that animals eat; they accumulate in animal fats and then they end up accumulating in human fat as we eat the meat and dairy products from the animals. In fact, food apparently accounts for 95 percent of human exposure to dioxin.

Medical Imaging Radiation

A 2006 report of the National Research Council of The National Academies concluded that there is evidence for a relationship between exposure to ionizing radiation and the development of cancer in humans.[26] As a result, the safety of radiation used in medical imaging especially is under scrutiny. Despite its great medical benefits, there is concern about potential radiation-related cancer risk.

CT scans, once rare, are now routine. One in 10 Americans undergo a CT scan every year, and many of them get more than one. This growth is a result of multiple factors, including a desire for early diagnoses, higher quality imaging technology, direct-to-consumer advertising and the financial interests of doctors and imaging centers. A 2009 National Cancer Institute study estimated that CT scans conducted in 2007 will cause a projected 29,000 excess cancer cases and 14,500 excess deaths over the lifetime of those exposed.[27]

The Institute of Medicine concluded that radiation from medical imaging in addition to hormone therapy, the use of which has substantially declined in the last decade, were the leading environmental causes of breast cancer and advised that women reduce their exposure to unnecessary CT scans.[28]

According to the calculations of cardiologist Rita Redberg and radiologist Rebecca Smith-Bindman at the University of California San Francisco Medical Center, unless we change our current practices, 3 to 5 percent of all future cancers may result from exposure to medical imaging. Given the many scans performed over the last several years, a reasonable estimate of excess lifetime cancers would be in the hundreds of thousands.[29]

In 2012, the American Association of Physicists in Medicine rolled out standardized procedures for adult CT exams.[30] What's more, the American College of Radiology sets limits for radiation doses and evaluates image quality. So far researchers have discovered that they can diagnose certain abnormal growths in the lungs and perform routine chest exams with about 75 percent less radiation than usual—a strategy Massachusetts General Hospital has since adopted. No matter how much clinicians lower the levels of radiation used in individual CT exams, however, a problem remains. Many people still receive unnecessary CT scans and, along with them, unneeded doses of radiation.

Bruce Hillman of the University of Virginia and other researchers are concerned that emergency room physicians in particular order too many CT scans in order to make quick decisions in high-pressure situations. "The jury is still out on whether there is a small cancer risk," said Donald Frush, chief of pediatric radiology at Duke University Medical Center.

"But the safest thing is to assume that no amount of radiation is safe. And if we find out in 20 years that a little bit was not harmful, then what did we lose by trying to minimize the dose?"

The public is largely unaware of the lifetime medical radiation and cancer risk radiation doses delivered by CT, positron emission tomography (PET scans) and other examinations that involve ionizing radiation. If patients were more aware of the cancer risk that can accrue with cumulative medical radiation exposure, they might be more likely to raise this issue with their physicians. Doctors then may suggest alternatives that do not involve radiation (e.g., blood tests, magnetic resonance imaging and ultrasound) but still yield sufficient diagnostic information. A recently initiated international project would facilitate such doctor-patient discussions by developing "smart cards" on which all radiation doses received by an individual are recorded.[31]

Radiofrequency Fields (Cell Phones)

The International Agency for Research on Cancer, a component of the World Health Organization, has recently classified radiofrequency fields as "possibly carcinogenic to humans." This is based on limited evidence from human and animal studies of its effects on immune system function, gene and protein expression, cell signaling, oxidative stress, apoptosis and the blood-brain barrier.

A large prospective cohort study of cell phone use and its possible long-term health effects was launched in Europe in March 2010. This study, known as COSMOS, has enrolled approximately 290,000 cell phone users 18 years and older to date and will follow them for 20 to 30 years.[32]

Laboratory Tests for Cancer

Finding laboratory tests that indicate neoplastic activity or the actual presence of cancer cells is one of the most promising approaches for detecting early-stage malignant and even premalignant lesions and following the progress of cancer.

Complete blood counts are used to diagnose blood cancers, such as leukemia. These tests detect differences in the number, size and maturity of white and red blood cells. People with leukemia typically have an elevated number of abnormal white blood cells that can be distinguished from normal white blood cells.

The PSA test for prostate cancer has proved to be controversial so that the 2013 Prostate Cancer World Congress recommended a baseline test at the age of 40 with screening for men between 50 and 69. Better screening tests are being explored in order to minimize the unnecessary and sometimes harmful effects of radiation and surgical treatments that are used for prostate lesions detected by biopsies.[33] Until a better test is found, the PSA remains widely used.

Dr. Victor Velculescu at the Johns Hopkins Kimmel Cancer Center has used data from the whole genome sequencing of cancer patients to develop individualized blood tests that may help physicians tailor patients' treatments.[34] The genome-based blood tests, believed to be the first of their kind, may be used to monitor tumor levels after therapy and determine cancer recurrence. Other examples of markers that can be used include:

- CA (cancer antigen) 15.3: used to find breast and ovarian cancers;
- TRU-QUANT and CA 27.29: may mean that breast cancer is present;
- CEA (carcinoembryonic antigen): a marker for the presence of colon, lung and liver cancers. This marker may be used to determine if breast cancer has traveled to other areas of the body;
- calcitonin for medullary thyroid cancer;
- alpha-fetoprotein (AFP) for liver cancer;
- human chorionic gonadotropin (HCG) for germ cell tumors, such as testicular cancer and ovarian cancer;
- circulating tumor cells: cells that break off from the cancer and move into the blood stream. High circulating tumor cell counts indicate that the cancer is growing. The CellSearch test has been approved by the Food and Drug Administration to monitor

circulating tumor cells in patients diagnosed with metastatic breast, colorectal and prostate cancer. Although not intended to replace imaging, results supplement imaging in the assessment of disease progression in patients with metastatic cancer.

Cancer is related to overall inflammation, which is reflected in c-reactive protein (CRP) levels that can be measured in the blood. Optimal CRP levels are under 0.55 mg/L in men and 1.0 mg/L in women. Heavier individuals usually have higher CRP levels since abdominal fat provides fertile ground for the over-production of pro-inflammatory cytokines that cause CRP to increase. Obese individuals often are in a chronic inflammatory state that increases their risk for all degenerative diseases and cancer.

Plasma DNA levels are significantly elevated in patients with esophageal cancer and return to normal levels following complete surgical removal of the cancer.[35] Persistently elevated blood DNA levels after surgery or levels that rise on follow-up indicate residual or recurrent cancer. The plasma DNA test also is used in breast cancer and may have broader applications.

A new blood test, developed at SRI Biosciences, can detect metastasizing cancer early. The test, called Fiber-optic Array Scanning Technology, or FASTcell, offers a high degree of sensitivity.[36] The test can scan 25-26 million cells in a minute, allowing surveying all of the blood cells in a sample. It has been compared to finding a single star in a whole constellation.

The ENOX2 protein species in the blood is unique for malignant cancer cells. These proteins are highly sensitive markers for early detection in both primary and recurrent cancer. The ONCOblot® detects their presence. The test is approved by Clinical Laboratory Improvement Amendments and the College of American Pathologists and was made available in January of 2013.[37]

A personalized blood test that can tell whether a patient's cancer has spread or come back has been found at Johns Hopkins University by Dr. Bert Vogelstein and colleagues. They found that circulating tumor DNA (ctDNA) measurements could be used to reliably monitor tumor dynamics in subjects with cancer who were undergoing surgery or chemotherapy.[38]

An international team of researchers, led by the Institute of Photonic Sciences in Barcelona, Spain, has developed a "lab-on-a-chip" platform capable of detecting very low concentrations of protein cancer markers in the blood, using the latest advances in plasmonics, nano-fabrication, microfluids and surface chemistry. Currently, most cancers are detected when a tumor is already composed of millions of cancer cells, and the disease is starting to advance into a more mature phase. The new device enables diagnosis of the disease in its earliest stages.[39]

Stool tests are being developed as an alternative to a colonoscopy in detecting colon-rectal cancer. One of them is Cologuard, a stool DNA test.[40]

Breath Tests for Cancer

Thanks to their keen noses, trained dogs are able to identify breath samples from patients with lung cancer with 98 percent accuracy.[41] Taking inspiration from our four-legged friends, a Mountain View California-based company called Metabolomx has completed a clinical trial that utilizes a breathalyzer to test for lung cancer—similar to how a dog would—with 83 percent accuracy. It works by using a proprietary colorimetric sensor array of reactants that change color depending on the compound with which it comes into contact. Patients are simply required to breathe into the machine for 5 minutes, which then removes both moisture and bacteria, allowing the reactants to detect potentially harmful compounds. This test is relatively inexpensive, costing about $75 to administer. Trials suggest that the device can not only tell that lung cancer is present, but what type of cancer it is.

Chemical Analysis of Tissues

At the present time the most effective and efficient way of examining body tissues and cells is through viewing them through microscopes.

Imperial College London researchers have developed a new method for analyzing biological samples based on their chemical makeup that could transform the way medical scientists examine diseased tissue.[42]

Conclusion

By applying the public health approach to cancer, oncology employs primary prevention through identifying genetic and environmental factors that contribute to developing neoplasia, such as smoking, air pollution and food additives. Secondary prevention is employed in treatments that aim to stop neoplasia. Tertiary prevention is managing the course of cancer.

Caring for patients with cancer and restoring them to health require the wide-ranging collaboration of diagnosticians, therapists and support services. Unfortunately, for most patients, care remains fragmented and uncoordinated. All stakeholders—including patients, clinicians, private and government payers and the pharmaceutical and device industries—need to work together to address improving cancer care.

The team model is growing across the medical-research community. For investigators, it means changes in the way careers are developed, the way data—and especially credit for achievement—are shared. For institutions, team research means changes in contracts, compensation, titles and intellectual property ownership. For pharmaceutical companies, it means restructuring the way experimental drugs are allocated and clinical trials are conducted.

There are a number of factors that we know stimulate neoplasia. Foremost among them are ultraviolet light, smoking, asbestos, obesity, nuclear radiation, chemical and particulate air and water pollution and medical imaging radiation. Toxic materials that accumulate in particular environments can cause clusters of people with cancer.

Finding blood tests that indicate neoplastic activity or the actual presence of cancer cells is one of the most promising approaches for detecting early-stage malignant or even premalignant lesions and following the progress of cancer.

Chapter Sixteen

How Can We Win the War on Cancer?

*The book concludes with a charge to become an
advocate for truly winning the War on Cancer
with suggestions about what you can do.*

We cannot improve cancer care without improving our health care system in general. Conversely, improving cancer care would markedly improve health care, since one of the most significant aspects of health care that obviously needs to change is our approach to cancer.

In January 2013, the National Research Council and the Institute of Medicine issued *U.S. Health in International Perspective: Shorter Lives, Poorer Health*—a stunning depiction of how, over the past four decades, the comparative health status of Americans has declined.[1] Strikingly, the report applied a term, commonly used to describe the relative deprivation of certain social groups, to the United States as a whole: the "U.S. health disadvantage."

The American Society of Clinical Oncology pointed out in 2014 that the demand for cancer prevention, screening and treatment services is growing rapidly.[2]

By 2030, the number of new cancer cases in the United States will increase by 45 percent, and cancer will become the nation's leading cause of death, largely as a result of the aging of the nation's population. At the same time, the number of cancer survivors, now almost 13.7 million, will continue to grow. Many of these individuals will require significant, ongoing care.

Access to quality cancer care remains uneven. Millions of people with cancer lack access to quality medical care, and rates of access to care are disproportionately lower for African Americans and Latinos. Today, one quarter of uninsured individuals forego care because of cost, and those without a regular source of care are less likely to receive cancer screening.

The Patient Protection and Affordable Care Act (ACA) is expected to provide millions more Americans with health insurance coverage in the coming years, but millions of Americans are expected to remain uninsured even after the ACA is implemented.

Soaring costs have created an urgent need to improve the value of patient care. While costs are rising throughout the healthcare system, the trend is especially pronounced in cancer care annual costs that are projected to rise from $104 billion in 2006 to more than $173 billion in 2020. This increase is a result of many factors, including the cost of many new cancer therapies. Access to high-quality cancer care will be sustained and expanded only if we address these rising costs, including the use of unnecessary or ineffective tests and treatments.

Researchers at Columbia University's Mailman School of Public Health call for a National Commission on the Health of Americans to hold public hearings and determine vigorous steps that must be taken to improve not just the health care of those at the bottom but the health care of Americans as a whole.[3] There is strong evidence for action beyond interventions at the individual level. It's time to reverse a course of events at least four decades in the making that have put the United States last among comparable nations in health care.

There is reason to hope that the focus of cancer research and treatment will be guided by the visions of the American Society of Clinical Oncology and the Director of the National Cancer Institute, Dr. Harold Varmus, to change the "conversation" from a search for and destroy cancer cells focus to preventing and stopping the underlying processes that produce them.[4]

Up to 50 percent of cancer deaths are preventable by making positive lifestyle changes. Quitting smoking, losing weight if you're overweight, exercising and eating nutritious foods clearly lower your cancer risk significantly.

Still, the financial incentives of the cancer culture and industries responsible for polluting our environment are not conducive to preventing and eradicating cancer. The ideas that "cancer is an evolutionary process destined to ensure the survival of the fittest" and that cancer is inevitable also contribute to a sense of hopelessness. For these reasons, strong public advocacy, including yours, will be required to focus research and treatment on designing effective treatments, reducing environmental pollution and promoting healthy life styles.

<u>Private Charities</u>

In the private sector you need to know what cancer charities are doing with the money they receive and how much of it is going into meaningful research.

In 2013 the Charity Navigator reviewed the financial health of over two dozen of the largest charities working to fight and prevent breast cancer in America.[5] Although these charities have been very successful in generating support, together raising nearly $1.7 billion annually in contributions, the disparity in their financial transparency and effectiveness is enormous.

The good news is that several of these charities efficiently utilize donations to pursue their mission. However, others will astound donors with their inefficient operations and low marks for accountability & transparency. For example, one charity spends less than 2% of its budget on fund raising expenses, while another spends nearly 98%. Many of these charities spend at least 80% of their budgets on programs and services, while four spend less than 50%. And while more than half of them earn high ratings for their commitment to accountability & transparency, three of them earn 0-stars and two earn just 1-star in this area.

Before contributing to any charity, it's advisable to look into their management through organizations that evaluate their transparency and effectiveness, such as the Charity Navigator, Greatnonprofits and the BBB Wise Giving Alliance.

The Public Sector

In *Clinical Cancer Advances 2013: Annual Report on Progress Against Cancer* by the American Society of Clinical Oncology,[6] President Clifford A. Hudis said that "our position as a world leader in advancing medical knowledge and our ability to attract the most promising and talented investigators are now threatened by an acute problem. Federal funding for cancer research has steadily eroded over the past decade, and only 15% of the ever-shrinking budget is actually spent on clinical trials. This dismal reality threatens the pace of progress against cancer and undermines our ability to address the continuing needs of our patients."

The American Society of Clinical Oncology is providing the scientific and clinical leadership needed. Dr. Harold Varmus, Director of the National Cancer Institute, is committed to providing the vision and the funding directions that are needed to "change the conversation" about cancer.

In his book *Reinventing American Health Care: How the Affordable Care Act will Improve our Terribly Complex, Blatantly Unjust, Outrageously Expensive, Grossly Inefficient, Error Prone System*, Dr. Ezekiel Emanuel, professor of medical ethics and health policy at the University of Pennsylvania, sorts out the complexities of the background, development, political wrangling and legal journey of the Affordable Care Act and describes its potential for improving our health care system.[7]

In the public sector we all need to put pressure on our elected representatives to fund sensible research. Those of us who are receiving cancer treatment now—over 13.7 million—and our caregivers have a compelling incentive to become politically active. We must inform the rest of the nation that one in three of us will ultimately die from cancer and that the costs of cancer care affect all of us. Our environment and life styles are the principal causes of cancer.[8] Inherited genetic factors play a minor role most types of cancer.

Advocacy in cancer care and prevention has played a major role in improving cancer control and care all over the world.[9] Organizations devoted to specific forms of cancer have moved from local, regional and national to global coalitions and federations. They all stress the need for persons with cancer and their caregivers to be involved in the challenges of cancer care and its improvement at policy and resource development levels. Bringing about the improvement of cancer requires public demand and lobbying by individuals and advocacy organizations.

In fact, there is no greater potential constituency for producing the political will for change than the War on Cancer can muster if properly directed. "Walk for cancer," "run for cancer," "cycle for cancer" are slogans that could generate popular support for changing the focus from killing cancer cells to preventing and stopping neoplasia. The desire is there. The energy is there. The money is there. What's missing is dedicated and effective leadership to make the War on Cancer one that we can win. Good intentions and appeals to charitable impulses are not enough.

What You and I Can Do

My effort to change the cancer care system is evident in this book. I also take every chance I have to inform others about the way that cancer affects all of us. Your own interests, talents and contacts offer opportunities to share your personal experience and efforts as well.

If you are so inclined and able, participating in any of the organizations mentioned in this book will offer you chances to both inform others and to learn more about cancer yourself. If you are reluctant to talk about your own experiences, please think twice. Again, everyone is affected by cancer, and your disclosures may help others to talk about their experiences.

At the very least, bear in mind that you have elected representatives who are more interested in input from their constituents than most people realize. Your most direct connection is with your Congressional

Representative and Senator. These persons will respond to your communication about your personal situation and about your desire to focus more federal attention on cancer care and research. You can send that person copies of articles or books that express your views, and, if possible, direct attention to relevant current issues. You can make contact with your Representative through http://www.house.gov/representatives/find/ and your Senator through http://www.senate.gov/general/contact_information/senators_cfm.cfm.

If you mention your interest in advocacy for winning the War on Cancer to your doctors, they may well have more specific suggestions for you.

Conclusion

Once again, the traditional focus on killing cancer cells puts the cart before the horse and explains why our conventional treatment of different forms of cancer has and will continue to lead us to a dead end in the War on Cancer.

We have lost decades of potential progress against cancer. Public understanding of the situation and pressure for change is needed to point cancer research and care in a preventive and curative direction by supporting and funding the initiatives of the American Association of Clinical Oncology and the Director of the National Cancer Institute that focus on the process through which cancer cells develop—neoplasia.

It is up to Congress to intelligently and effectively provide adequate funding that is not dictated by the financial incentives of industry lobbyists and the unrealistic regulation and conduct of clinical trials but by the goal of preventing and treating neoplasia.

References

Acknowledgements

1. a) American Society of Clinical Oncology (2011) *Accelerating Progress Against Cancer: ASCO's Blueprint for Transforming Clinical and Translational Cancer Research*. Alexandria, Virginia: American Society of Clinical Oncology; b) http://www.asco.org/sites/default/files/shapingfuture-lowres.pdf.
2. a) Faguet, Guy B. (2008) *The War on Cancer: An Anatomy of Failure, A Blueprint for the Future*. Springer; b) Faguet, Guy B. (2014) *The Conquest of Cancer*. Dordrecht, The Netherlands: Springer.
3. Sporn, Michael (2011) Perspective: The big C - for Chemoprevention. *Nature*. 471 (7339): S10-1.
4. Mukherjee, Siddhartha (2010) *The Emperor of All Maladies: A Biography of Cancer*. New York: Scribner.
5. Shapin, Steven (2010) Cancer World: The Making of a Modern Disease. *The New Yorker*. November 8.
6. Seyfried, Thomas (2012) *Cancer as a Metabolic Disease: On the Origin, Management, and Prevention of Cancer*. New York: Wiley & Son.
7. Leaf, Clifton (2004) Why We're Losing the War on Cancer. *Fortune*. March 22.
8. Leaf, Clifton (2013) *The Truth in Small Doses: Why We're Losing the War on Cancer-and How to Win It*. New York: Simon and Schuster.
9. Saporito, Bill with Park, Alice (2013) The Conspiracy To End Cancer. *Time*. April 1.
10. George Johnson (2013) *The Cancer Chronicles: Unlocking Medicine's Deepest Mystery*. New York: Knopf.

Chapter Two - Conventional Cancer Treatment

1. a) Vartholomeos, P. & Mavroidis, C. (2012) In Silico Studies of Magnetic Microparticle Aggregations in Fluid Environments for MRI-Guided Drug

Delivery. *IEEE Transactions on Biomedical Engineering.* 59 (11): 3028–3038; b) Inanc, Ortac, et al. (2014) Dual-Porosity Hollow Nanoparticles for the Immunoprotection and Delivery of Nonhuman Enzymes. *Nano Letters.* 14 (6): 3023–3032. c) http://www.scientificamerican.com/magazine/sa/2014/07-01/, Volume 311, No. 1.

2. Albergotti, R. & O'Connell, V. (2013) *Wheelman: Lance Armstrong, the Tour de France, and the Greatest Sports Conspiracy Ever.* New York: Gotham.

3. Emanuel, E. J. (2013) A Plan To Fix Cancer Care. *The New York Times.* March 23; http://opinionator.blogs.nytimes.com/2013/03/23/a-plan-to-fix-cancer-care/

4. American Society of Clinical Oncology (2011) *Accelerating Progress Against Cancer: ASCO's Blueprint for Transforming Clinical and Translational Cancer Research.* Alexandria, Virginia: American Society of Clinical Oncology.

5. Nazaryan, A. (2013) World War Cancer. *The New Yorker.* July 1, 2013.

6. Leaf, Clifton (2013) *The Truth in Small Doses: Why We're Losing the War on Cancer-and How to Win It.* New York: Simon and Schuster.

7. Davis, J. S. & Wu, X. (2012) Current state and future challenges of chemoprevention. *Discovery Medicine* (72): 385-90.

8. Hayes, Julie H., et al. (2013) Observation versus initial treatment for men with localized, low-risk prostate cancer: a cost-effectiveness analysis. *Annals of Internal Medicine.* 158 (12): 853-860.

9. U.S. Preventive Services Task Force. (2009) Screening for breast cancer: U.S. Preventive Services Task Force Recommendation Statement. *Annals of Internal Medicine.* 151: 716-726.

10. Miller, Anthony B., et al. (2014) Twenty-five-year follow-up for breast cancer incidence and mortality of the Canadian National Breast Screening Study: randomized screening trial. *British Medical Journal.* 348: g366 doi: 10.1136/bmj.g366.

11. a) Parker-Pope, Tara (2013) Scientists Seek to Rein In Diagnoses of Cancer. *The New York Times.* July 30, p. 1A; b) Esserman, Laura J., et al. (2013) Overdiagnosis and Overtreatment in Cancer: An Opportunity for Improvement. *Journal of the American Medical Association.* 310 (8): 797-798.

12. Kaiser, Jocelyn (2013) Varmus's Second Act. *Science.* 342: 416-419.

13. Levit, Laura A., et al. (2013) *Delivering High-Quality Cancer Care: Charting a New Course for a System in Crisis.* Washington, DC: The National Academies Press.

14. Hough, Douglas E. (2013) *Irrationality in Health Care: What Behavioral Economics Reveals About What We Do and Why.* Stanford, CA: Stanford University Press.

15. American Cancer Institute (2013) *Last Days of Life (PDQ).* Washington, DC: National Cancer Institute.

16. http://qopi.asco.org/program.html.
17. Butow, Phyllis & Baille, Walter F. (2012) Communication in Cancer Care: A Cultural Perspective. In Grassi, Luigi & Riba, Michelle. *Clinical Psycho-oncology: An International Perspective*. New York: Wiley-Blackwell.

Chapter Three - Navigating the Cancer Care System

1. http://www.choosingwisely.org/doctor-patient-lists/.
2. http://www.himssehra.org/ASP/index.asp.
3. http://www.altossolutions.com/SeeYourChart.htm.
4. http://www.epic.com/software-phr.php.
5. a) http://en.wikipedia.org/wiki/Personal_health_record; b) My Medical http://mymedicalapp.com/; b) Personal Portable Electronic Medical Records; and c) http://www.personalportableelectronicmedicalrecords.com/Home.html.
6. http://en.wikipedia.org/wiki/Personal_health_record.
7. http://www.cancer.net/survivorship/asco-cancer-treatment-summaries.
8. http://www.cancer.net/survivorship/survivorship-next-steps-take-after-treatment
9. http://www.accessmyrecords.com/.
10. Ubel, Peter A. (2013) *Critical Decisions: How You and Your Doctor Can Make the Right Medical Choices Together*. New York: HarperOne.
11. Sullivan, Paul (2013) Planning a Future in the Face of Terminal Illness. *The New York Times*. November 20, p. F2.
12. Taha, Nadia (2013) Medicaid Help Without Falling into Poverty. *The New York Times*. November 19, p. F3.
13. a) www.medicaid.gov; b) www.va.gov.
14. Goldman, Bob (2013) For Those at Death's Door, a Case for 'Life Panels'. *The New York Times*. November 19, p. F8.
15. a) *Virtual Mentor* (2014) 16 (5): 357-358; b) Institute of Medicine (2014) *Dying in America: Improving Quality and Honoring Individual Preferences Near the End of Life*. Washington, DC: Institute of Medicine.
16. http://www.cancer.org/cancer/bookstore/view-all-books.
17. http://www.cancer.gov/cancertopics/cancerlibrary.
18. http://www.apos-society.org.
19. http://www.cancer.net/.
20. Ubel, Peter (2013) *Critical Decisions: How You and Your Doctor Can Make the Right Medical Choices Together*. New York: HarperOne.

21. Vincent, Lorie L. & Vincent, Mark L. (2011) *Fighting Disease, Not Death: Finding a Way Through Lifelong Struggle.* Dog Ear Publishing.

22. Holmes, Greg & Roth, Katherine (2013) *The Good Fight: A Story of Cancer, Love, and Triumph.* Paradox Press.

23. Madhulika Sikka (2014) *A Breast Cancer Alphabet.* New York: Crown Publishing Group

24. http://www.patientadvocatetraining.com/.

25. Palmieri, Carlo, Bird, Esther & Simcock, Richard (Eds.) (2013) *ABC of Cancer Care (ABC Series).* New York: Wiley Blackwell.

26. Alternative Cancer Research Institute (2011) *The Complete Guide to Alternative Cancer Treatment.* Lexington, VA: Online Publishing and Marketing.

Chapter Four – Background for Understanding Cancer

1. Shapin, Steven (2010) Cancer World: The Making of a Modern Disease. *The New Yorker.* November 8.

2. Buchan, William (1769) *Domestic Medicine. Or, A Treatise on the Prevention and Cure of Diseases by Regimen and Simple Medicines.* London: A. Strahan.

3. Mukherjee, Siddhartha (2010) *The Emperor of All Maladies: A Biography of Cancer.* New York: Scribner.

4. Kleinman, Arthur (1989) *The Illness Narrative: Suffering, Healing, and the Human Condition.* NewYork: Basic Books.

5. Fenner, Frank (2008) Frank Macfarlane Burnet as I Knew Him. *Immunology and Cell Biology.* 86: 22-23.

6. Shapin, Steven (2010) Cancer World: The Making of a Modern Disease. *The New Yorker.* November 8.

7. Thomas, Lewis (1982) On immunosurveillance in human cancer. *Yale Journal of Biology and Medicine.* 55 (3-4): 329–333.

8. *Journal of the National Cancer Institute* (1990) 82 (3): 176-178.)

9. Cell Press (2004) The Immunobiology Review of Cancer Immunosurveillance and Immunoediting. *Immunity.* 21: 137–148.

10. Human Genome Project (2004) *European Journal of Cancer.* 40 (17): 2537-43.

11. Faguet, Guy, B. (2008) *The War on Cancer: An Anatomy of Failure.* Dordrecht, The Netherlands: Springer.

12. American Cancer Society (2013) *Cancer Facts & Figures 2013.* Atlanta: American Cancer Society.

13. op. cit. Faguet, Guy B.

14. Leaf, Clifton (2013) *The Truth in Small Doses: Why We're Losing the War on Cancer-and How to Win It.* New York: Simon and Schuster.

15. Leaf, Clifton (2004) Why We're Losing the War On Cancer. *Fortune.* March 22, 2004.

16. Remarks of President Barack Obama to Joint Session of Congress, Tuesday, February 24th, 2009.

17. Cauvin, Henrie E. (2000) Cancer Researcher in South Africa Who Falsified Data Is Fired. *The New York Times.* March 11.

18. Williams, Mary Elizabeth (2013) Is there too much breast cancer "awareness"? *Salon.* April 25.

19. Orenstein, Peggy (2013) The Problem with Pink: Our Feel-Good War on Breast Cancer. *The New York Times Magazine.* April 28, pp. 37-71.

Chapter Five - How Cancer Cells Form and Multiply

1. Sharma, Monika, et al. (2013) DNA Bending Propensity in the Presence of Base Mismatches: Implications for DNA Repair. *Journal of Physical Chemistry.* 117: 6194-6205.

2. Gasser, S. & Raulet, D. H. (2006) The DNA damage response arouses the immune system. *Cancer Research.* 66 (8): 3959-62.

3. Hanahan, D. & Weinberg, R. A. (2011) Hallmarks of Cancer: The Next Generation. *Cell.* 144 (5): 646-74.

4. National Cancer Institute. *Understanding Cancer Series: Neoplasia.* Washington, DC: National Cancer Institute.

5. Piccolo, Stefano (2014) Twists of Fate. *Scientific American.* 311 (4): 75-81.

6. Byun, S., et al. (2013) Characterizing deformability and surface friction of cancer cells. *Proceedings of the National Academy of Sciences USA.* 110: 7580–5.

7. a) Kong, A. T. (2014) Inflammation, Oxidative Stress, and Cancer: Dietary Approaches for Cancer Prevention. Boca Raton, FL: CRC Press; b) U.S. Department of Health and Human Services (2011) *12th Report on Carcinogens.*

8. a) Moore, Patrick S. & Chang, Yuan (2010) Why do viruses cause cancer? Highlights of the first century of human tumour virology. *Cancer.* 10: 878-889; b) Butel, Janet S. (1999) Viral carcinogenesis: revelation of molecular mechanisms and etiology of human disease. *Journal of Carcinogensis.* 21 (3): 405-426; c) zur Hausen, H. (1991) Viruses in human cancers. *Science.* 254 (5035): 1167–73.

9. Omberg, Larsson, et al. (2013) Enabling transparent and collaborative computational analysis of 12 tumor types within The Cancer Genome Atlas. *Nature Genetics.* 45: 1121–1126.

10. http://io9.com/5975002/james-watson-says-antioxidants-may-actually-be-causing-cancer.

11. Vogelstein, Bert, et al. (2013) Cancer Genome Landscapes. *Science*. 339 (6127): 1546-1558.

12. http://www.stopcancerfund.org/in-the-news/angelina-jolies-decision/.

13. a) Kaipparettu B. A., et al. (2013) Crosstalk from non-cancerous mitochondria can inhibit tumor properties of metastatic cells by suppressing oncogenic pathways. *PLoS One*. 8, e61747; b) Elliott R. L., et al. (2012) Mitochondria organelle transplantation: introduction of normal epithelial mitochondria into human cancer cells inhibits proliferation and increases drug sensitivity. *Breast Cancer Research and Treatment*. 136: 347–354.

14. Warburg, Otto (1930) *Metabolism of Tumours*. London: Constable.

15. Christofferson, T. (2013) What is the origin of cancer? http://robbwolf.com/2013.

16. Seyfried, Thomas (2012) *Cancer as a Metabolic Disease: On the Origin, Management, and Prevention of Cancer*. New York: Wiley & Son.

17. Pedersen, Peter (2007) Warburg, me and Hexokinase 2: Multiple discoveries of key molecular events underlying one of cancers' most common phenotypes, the "Warburg Effect". *Journal of Bioenergetics and Biomembranes*. 39: 211–222.

18. Pedersen, Peter (2012) Mitochondria in relation to cancer metastasis: introduction to a mini-review series. *Journal of Bioenergetics and Biomembranes*. 44: 615–617.

19. Mathupala, Saroj P., et al. (2009) Hexokinase-2 bound to mitochondria: Cancer's stygian link to the "Warburg effect" and a pivotal target for effective therapy. *Seminars in Cancer Biology*. 19: 17–24.

20. Ko, Y. H., et al. (2001) *Cancer Letters*. 173: 83–91.

21. (a) Sloan, Erica K., et al. (2010) The Sympathetic Nervous System Induces a Metastatic Switch in Primary Breast Cancer. *Cancer Research*. 70 (18): 7042–52; b) Sood, Anil K., et al. (2010) Adrenergic modulation of focal adhesion kinase protects human ovarian cancer cells from anoikis. *Journal of Clinical Investigation*. 120 (5):1515-1523; c) Wolford, Chris C., et al. (2013) Transcription factor ATF3 links host adaptive response to breast cancer metastasis. *Journal of Clinical Investigation*. 123 (7): 2893-2906.

22. Hemminki, K., et al. (2012) Effect of autoimmune diseases on risk and survival in female cancers. *Gynecologic Oncology*. 127 (1):180-185.

23. Derra, Skip (2013) Exposing cancer's deep evolutionary roots. *Research Matters*. http://researchmatters.asu.edu/stories/cancer-theory-evolutionary-roots-2708#sthash.UjkRGnnP.dpuf.

24. a) Cole, L. A. (2012) HCG, the wonder of today's science. *Reproductive Bioliology and Endocrinolology*. 10: 24. b) Wieczorek, Maciej, et al. (2008)

Silencing of Wnt-1 by siRNA induces apoptosis of MCF-7 human breast cancer cells. *Cancer Biology & Therapy.* 7 (2): 268-274; c) Goyeneche, A. A., et al. (2012) Mifepristone prevents repopulation of ovarian cancer cells escaping Cis-platin-paclitaxel therapy. *BMC Cancer.* 12: 200; d) Ligr, M., et al. (2012) Mifepristone inhibits GRβ coupled prostate cancer cell proliferation. *Journal of Urology.* 188 (3): 981-8.

25. Why Don't We Get Heart Cancer? *TIME.* September 8-15, 2014, p. 65.
26. Nakashima, R. A., Paggi, M. G., Pedersen, P. L. (1984) Contributions of glycolysis and oxidative phosphorylation to adenosine 5'-triphosphate production in AS-30D hepatoma cells. *Cancer Research.* 44 (12 Pt 1): 5702-6.
27. http://physicsworld.com/cws/article/indepth/2013/jul/01/exposing-cancers-deep-evolutionary-roots.

Chapter Six - Cancer Research

1. American Society of Clinical Oncology (2011) *Accelerating Progress Against Cancer: ASCO's Blueprint for Transforming Clinical and Translational Cancer Research.* Alexandria, Virginia: American Society of Clinical Oncology.
2. Ellis, Lee M., et al. (2104) American Society of Clinical Oncology Perspective: Raising the Bar for Clinical Trials by Meaningful Outcomes. *Journal of Clinical Oncology.* 32 (12): 1277-1280.
3. How Science Goes Wrong. *The Economist.* October 19, 2013, p. 13.
4. Editorial (2013) Reducing our irreproducibility. *Nature.* 496: 398.)
5. a) Ioannidis, John P. A. (2005) Contradicted and Initially Stronger Effects in Highly Cited Clinical Research. *Journal of the American Medical Association.* 294 (2): 218-228; b) Ioannidis, John P. A. (2005) Why Most Published Research Findings Are False. *Plos-Medicine.* August 30.
6. Kaiser, Jocelyn (2013) Varmus's Second Act. *Science.* 342: 416-419.
7. Pennisi, Elizabeth (2013) Steering Cancer Genomics into the Fast Lane. *Science.* 339 (6127): 1540-1542.
8. *Science* (2006) 15 September, p. 1553.
9. a) Ley, T. J., et al. (2008) DNA sequencing of a cytogenetically normal acute myeloid leukaemia genome. *Nature.* 456 (7218): 66-72; b) http://www.mskcc.org/cancer-care/trial/13-154.
10. Zhang J., et al. (2012) The genetic basis of early T-cell precursor acute lymphoblastic leukaemia. *Nature.* 481 (7380): 157-63.
11. Kaiser, Jocelyn (2013) The Downside of Diversity. *Science.* 339: 1543-154.
12. Kiberstis, Paula & Roberts, Leslie (2014) A Race Still Unfinished. *Science.* 343: 1451.

13. King, Mary-Clair (2014) "The Race" to Clone BRCA1. *Science*. 343: 1462-1465.

14. Kean, Sam (2104) The 'Other' Breast Cancer Genes. *Science*. 343: 1459.

15. Hoadley, Katherine A. (2014) Multiplatform Analysis of 12 Cancer Types Reveals Molecular Classification within and across Tissues of Origin. *Cell*. 158 (4): 929–944.

16. Ross, Theodora (2014) Cancer and the Secrets of Your Genes. *The New York Times*. August 16.

17. Leaf, Clifton (2013) *The Truth in Small Doses: Why We're Losing the War on Cancer-and How to Win It*. New York: Simon and Schuster.

18. NCI Press Release (08/08/2013): NIH scientists visualize how cancer chromosome abnormalities form in living cells. http://www.cancer.gov/newscenter/newsfromnci/2013/ChromosomeLivingCellsMisteli.

19. Marshall, John L. (2014) Silence the Mouse Model That Roared. *Medscape Oncology*. April 16.

20. Couzin-Frankel, Jennifer (2014) Chasing the Money. *Science*. 344 (6179): 24-25.

21. a) Leaf, Clifton (2004) Why We're Losing the War On Cancer. *Fortune*. March 22; b) http://budgettool.cancer.gov/budget-spending/funding-by-mechanism/research-project-grants/fiscal-year-2010/Funding.aspx.

22. Alberts, Bruce (2013) Am I wrong? *Science*. 339: 1252.

23. Cossins, Dan (2013) The Cancer-Test Kid. *The Scientist*. April 1. http://www.the-scientist.com/?articles.view/articleNo/34759/title/The-Cancer-Test-Kid/.

24. Anderson, Kent (2014) The Jack Andraka Story — Uncovering the Hidden Contradictions Behind a Science Folk Hero. http://scholarlykitchen.sspnet.org/2014/01/03/the-jack-andraka-story-uncovering-the-hidden-contradictions-of-an-oa-paragon/.

Chapter Seven - Testing Treatments

1. http://www.phrma.org/sites/default/files/1000/phrmamedicinesindevelopmentcancer2012.pdf.

2. *Fortune*. April 8, 2013. pp. 58-60.

3. Leaf, Clifton (2004) Why We're Losing the War On Cancer. *Fortune*. March 22.

4. Yoy, Avik S. A. (2012) *Stifling New Cures: The True Cost of Lengthy Clinical Drug Trials*. Project FDA Report No. 5. New York: Manhattan Institute for Policy Research.

5. Pharma & Healthcare (2013) The Cost of Creating a New Drug Now $5 Billion, Pushing Big Pharma To Change. *Forbes*. August 11.

6.   Leaf, Clifton (2013) *The Truth in Small Doses: Why We're Losing the War on Cancer-and How to Win It.* New York: Simon and Schuster.

7.   Huber, Peter W. (2013) *The Cure in the Code.* New York: Basic Books.

8.   http://www.pharmgkb.org/page/cpic.

9.   Beer, Tomasz M. (2013) Cancer Clinical Trials of Tomorrow. *The Scientist.* April 1.

10. Nass, Sharyl J. & Patlak, Margie (2013) *Implementing a National Cancer Clinical Trials System for the 21st Century.* Washington, DC: American Society of Clinical Oncology and Institute of Medicine Workshop.

11. Eichler, H. G., et al. (2012) Adaptive Licensing: Taking the Next Step in the Evolution of Drug Approval. *Clinical Pharmacology & Therapeutics.* 91 (3): 426-37.

12. ibid.

13. http://medicine.yale.edu/core/projects/yodap/index.aspx.

14. Sanghavi, Darshak (2013) The Pharmaceutical Hail Mary. *The New York Times Magazine.* October 19, pp. 40-43.

15. ibid.

16. The Editors (2014) Secret Clinical Trial Data to Go Public. *Scientific American.* 310 (6): 10.

17. Ellis, Lee M., et al. (2014) American Society of Clinical Oncology Perspective: Raising the Bar for Clinical Trials by Defining Clinically Meaningful Outcomes. *Journal of Clinical Oncology.* 32 (12): 1277-1283.

Chapter Eight - Changing the Way We Think About Cancer

1.   Saporito, Bill (2013) The Conspiracy to End Cancer: A team-based, cross-disciplinary approach to cancer research is upending tradition and delivering results faster. *Time.* April 01.

2.   a) Tisch, Roland, et al. (2012) Antibodies Reverse Type 1 Diabetes in New Immunotherapy Animal Study. *Diabetes.* 61 (11): 2871–2880; b) Zeng, Siswanto & Defu, et al. (2014) MHC-Mismatched Chimerism Is Required for Induction of Transplantation Tolerance in Autoimmune Nonobese Diabetic Recipients. *Journal of Immunology.* 193: 2005-2015.

3.   Sporn, Michael (2011) Perspective: The big C—for Chemoprevention. *Nature.* 471 (7339): S10-1.

4.   Leaf, Clifton (2013) *The Truth in Small Doses: Why We're Losing the War on Cancer-and How to Win It.* New York: Simon and Schuster.

5.   Ibid.

6. a) Banki, Farzaneh, et al. (2007) Plasma DNA as a Molecular Marker for Completeness of Resection and Recurrent Disease in Patients with Esophageal Cancer. *Archives of Surgery.* 142: 533-539; b) Shaw, J. A., et al. (2011) Circulating tumor cells and plasma DNA analysis in patients with indeterminate early or metastatic breast cancer. *Biomarkers in Medicine.* 5 (1): 87-91; c) Ghorbian, S. & Ardekani, Ali M. (2012) Non-Invasive Detection of Esophageal Cancer using Genetic Changes in Circulating Cell-Free DNA. *Avicenna Journal of Medical Biotechnology.* 4 (1): 3-13.

7. a) Ko, Y. H., et al. (2004) Advanced cancers: eradication in all cases using 3-bromopyruvate therapy to deplete ATP. *Biochemical and Biophysical Research Communications.* 324 (1): 269–75; b) Ko, Y. H., et al. (2012) A translational study "case report" on the small molecule "energy blocker" 3-bromopyruvate (3BP) as a potent anticancer agent: from bench side to bedside. *Journal of Bioenergetics and Biomembranes.* 44: 163–170; c) Pedersen, Peter L. (2012) 3-bromopyruvate (3BP) a fast acting, promising, powerful specific, and effective "small molecule" anti-cancer agent taken from labside to bedside: introduction to a special issue. *Journal of Bioenergy and Biomembranes.* 44: 1–6.

8. Dachsel, Justus C., et al. (2013) The Rho Guanine Nucleotide Exchange Factor Syx Regulates the Balance of Dia and ROCK Activities To Promote Polarized-Cancer-Cell Migration. *Molecular and Cellular Biology.* 13: 20-27-0800.

9. Friedman-Rudovsky, Jean (2013) Blue Scorpion Venom: Cuba's Miracle Drug. *Miami New Times.* April 18.

10. a) Keck, C. W. & Reed, G. A. (2012) The curious case of Cuba. *American Journal of Public Health.* 102 (8): e13-e22.2; b) Campion, Edward W. & Morrissey, Stephen (2013) A Different Model—Medical Care in Cuba. *New England Journal of Medicine.* 368: 297-299.

11. Davis, Rebecca (2013) Why Painting Tumors Could Make Brain Surgery Better. *Health News from NPR.* September 12, 2013.

Chapter Nine - Immunotherapy: Drawing upon Your Body's Resources

1. a) Hall, Stephen S. (1998) *A Commotion in the Blood: Life, Death, and the Immune System.* Owl Books; b) Coley, W. B. (1893) The Treatment of Malignant Tumors by Repeated Innoculations of Erysipelas: With a Report of Ten Original Cases. *American Journal of the Medical Sciences.* 10: 487–511.

2. Burnet, Frank M. (1957) Cancer—A Biological Approach: I. The Processes Of Control. II. The Significance of Somatic Mutation. *British Medical Journal.* 1 (5022): 779–786.

3. Olson, James S. (Ed.) (1989) *The History of Cancer: An Annotated Bibliography.* Westport, CT: Greenwood Press, p. 251.

4. a) Thomas, L. (1982) On immunosurveillance in human cancer. *Yale Journal of Biological Medicine.* 55: 329–333; b) Dunn, Gavin P., Old, Lloyd J. & Schreiber, Robert D. (2004) The Immunobiology of Cancer Immunosurveillance and Immunoediting. *Immunity.* 21: 137–148.

5. Leaf, Christopher (2013) *The Truth in Small Doses: Why We're Losing the War on Cancer-and How to Win It.* New York: Simon and Schuster.

6. Dunn, G. P., et al. (2004) The Immunobiology Review of Cancer Immunosurveillance and Immunoediting. *Immunity.* 21: 137–148.

7. Sporn, M. B. (2011) Perspective: The big C - for Chemoprevention. *Nature.* 471 (7339): S10-1.

8. May, Kenneth F., Jr., et al. (2011) Prostate Cancer Immunotherapy. *Clinical Cancer Research.* 17 (16): 5233–8.

9. a) Topalian, Suzzane (2013) American Association of Cancer Research Annual Meeting. Plenary Address, April 6; b) Huang, Yuhui (2014) Harnessing the immune system to cure cancer. *Translational Cancer Research.* 3 (3).

10. Coghlan, Andy (2006) Horror clinical trial in test tube recreation. *New Science Health.* 16:39.

11. Sylvester, R. J., et al. (2004). Intravesical Bacillus Calmette-Guerin reduces the risk of progression in patients with superficial bladder cancer: A meta-analysis of the published results of randomized clinical trials. *Journal of Urology.* 168 (5): 1964-1970.

12. www.novartis.com/newsroom/media-releases/en/2012/1631944.shtml

13. a) http://mb.cision.com/Public/3069/9393277/b82514490ac0538e.pdf; b) Marchione, Marilyn (2013) Gene therapy scores big wins against blood cancers. *The Associated Press.* Dec. 8.

14. a) http://www.uphs.upenn.edu/news/News_Releases/2014/04/aacr/; b) Bear, A. S., et al. (2012) Replication-Competent Retroviruses in Gene-Modified T Cells Used in Clinical Trials: Is It Time to Revise the Testing Requirements? *Molecular Therapy* 20: 246-249.

15. Vizcardo, Raul, et al. (2013) Regeneration of Human Tumor Antigen-Specific T Cells from iPSCs Derived from Mature CD8+ T Cells. *Cell Stem Cell.* 12 (1): 31–36.

16. UGA researchers use nanoparticles to fight cancer. *UGA Today.* September 16, 2013.

17. Topalian, Suzanne L., et al (2012) Safety, Activity, and Immune Correlates of Anti–PD-1 Antibody in Cancer. *New England Journal of Medicine.* 366: 2443-2454.

18. West, E. E., et al. (2013) PD-L1 blockade synergizes with IL-2 therapy in reinvigorating exhausted T cells. *Journal of Clinical Investigation.* 123 (6): 2604–2615.

19. Fong, Lawrence, et al. (2014) Improved Survival with T Cell Clonotype Stability After Anti–CTLA-4 Treatment in Cancer Patients. *Science Translational Medicine.* 6: (238): 238ra70.

20. Conner, Steve (2013) Exclusive: Cancer—A cure just got closer thanks to a tiny British company and the result could change the lives of millions. *The Independent.* July 28 (http://www.independent.co.uk.)

21. Weiner, L. M., et al. (2010) Mono-clonal antibodies: versatile platforms for cancer immunotherapy. Nature Reviews. *Immunology.* 10: 317-327.

22. Marrache, Sean, et al. (2013) Ex Vivo Programming of Dendritic Cells by Mitochondria-Targeted Nanoparticles to Produce Interferon-Gamma for Cancer Immunotherapy. *ACS Nano.* 7 (8): 7392–7402.

23. Rudnicka, Dominika, et al. (2013) Rituximab causes a polarization of B cells that augments its therapeutic function in NK-cell–mediated antibody-dependent cellular cytotoxicity. *Blood.* 121 (23): 4694-4702.

24. Cuji, Bing, et al. (2013) Targeting ROR1 Inhibits Epithelial–Mesenchymal Transition and Metastasis. *Cancer Research.* 73 (12): 3649–60.

25. Mart, Robert J., et al., (2013) BH3 helix-derived biophotonic nanoswitches regulate cytochrome c release in permeabilised cells. *Molecular BioSystems,* 2013, DOI: 10.1039/C3MB70246D.

26. a) http://www.lef.org/magazine/mag2012/nov2012_Innovative_Laser_Therapy_02.htm.
b) Adalsteinsson, O. (2012) Laser-Assisted Immunotherapy: A Novel Autologous Vaccine Strategy for Cancers with Solid Tumors Clinical Protocol #ISCA 0001 ed.: International Strategic Cancer Alliance; c) Chen, W. R., et al. (2006) Photoimmunotherapy for cancer treatment. *Journal of Environmental Pathology, Toxicology and Oncology.* 25 (1-2): 281-91; d) St Denisa, Tyler G., et al. (2011) Combination approaches to potentiate immune response after photodynamic therapy for cancer. *Photochemical and Photobiological Sciences.* 10 (5): 792–801.

27. a) Diane Tseng, Diane, et al. (2013) Anti-CD47 antibody–mediated phagocytosis of cancer by macrophages primes an effective antitumor T-cell response. *Proceedings of the National Academy of Sciences.* 110 (27) 11103-11108; b) Unanue, Emil R. (2013) Perspectives on anti-CD47 antibody treatment for experimental cancer. *Proceedings of the National Academy of Sciences.* 110 (27) 10886–10887.

28. Brody, Jane E. (2014) Outsmarting Breast Cancer. *The New York Times.* June 10, p. D7.

29. Cossins, Dan (2013) Exploring the Tumor Neighborhood. *The Scientist.* 27 (4) April 10.

30. Orenstein, Peggy (2013) The Problem with Pink: Our Feel-Good War on Breast Cancer. *The New York Times Magazine.* April 28, pp. 37-71.

31. May, Kenneth F., Jr., et al. (2011) Prostate Cancer Immunotherapy. *Clinical Cancer Research.* 17 (16): 5233–5238.

32. Barts Cancer Institute News (2013) Investigating the ovarian cancer microenvironment 25 April 2013.

33. Cossins, Dan (2013) Scientists highlighted research on the crucial role of the non-malignant cells that surround tumors in cancer initiation, growth, and response. *The Scientist.* April 10.

34. ibid.

35. http://www.salk.edu/news/pressrelease_details.php?press_id=2038

36. http://tmen.nci.nih.gov/Pages/Home.aspx.

37. Geddes, Linda (2009) Autoimmune disease cells harnessed to fight cancer. *New Scientist.* 18: 14-29.

38. Moira Wilke, Cailin, et al. (2011) Th17 cells in cancer: help or hindrance? *Carcinogenesis.* 32 (5): 643–649.

39. Holbreich, Mark, et al. (2012) The Prevalence of Asthma, Hay Fever and Allergic Sensitization in Amish Children. *Journal of Allergy and Clinical Immunology.* 129 (2) Supplement: AB130.

40. Romero, Pedro J., et al. (2012) Introducing the society for immunotherapy of cancer's new journal: *Journal for immunotherapy of Cancer.* 1 (1).

41. Overwijk, Willem, W., et al. (2013) Mining the mutanome: developing highly personalized Immunotherapies based on mutational analysis of tumors. *Journal for ImmunoTherapy of Cancer.* 1: 11.

42. Vatsan, Ramjay S., et al. (2013) Regulation of immunotherapeutic products for cancer and FDA's role in product development and clinical evaluation. *Journal for ImmunoTherapy of Cancer.* 1: 5.

43. Slikowski, Mark X. & Mellman, Ira (2013) Antibody Therapeutics in Cancer. *Science.* 341 (6151): 1192-1198.

Chapter Ten - Nutritional Therapy: Drawing upon Nature's Resources

1. Lineweaver, Charles H., Davies, Paul C. W., & Ruse, Michael (Eds.) (2013) *Complexity and the Arrow of Time.* Cambridge, UK: Cambridge University Press.

2. Gunnars, Kris (2012) Ketogenic Diets and Cancer–The Current State of Research. *Authority Nutrition.* December 19.

3. Warburg, O. (1930) *Metabolism of Tumours*. London: Constable.

4. Szent-Gyorgi, A., et al. (1963) Cancer Therapy: A Possible New Approach. *Science*. 140: 1391-1392.

5. Woods, M. W. & DuBuy, H. G. (1945) Cytoplasmic diseases and cancer. *Science*: 102: 591-593.

6. Modica-Napolitano, J. S. & Singh, K. K. (2002) Mitochondria as Targets for Detection and Treatment of Cancer. *Expert Reviews in Molecular Medicine*. 4 (9): 1-19.

7. Bonnet, S., et al. (2007) A Mitochondria-K+ Channel Axis Is Suppressed in Cancer and Its Normalization Promotes Apoptosis and Inhibits Cancer Growth. *Cancer Cell*. 11: 37–51.

8. a) Petit, P. X. & Kroemer, G. (1998) Mitochondrial regulation of apoptosis. In Singh, K. K. (ed.) *Mitochondrial DNA Mutations in Aging, Disease and Cancer*. Berlin: Springer-Veerlag, pp. 147-165; b) Plas, D. R., & Thompson, C. B. (2002) Cell metabolism in the regulation of programmed cell death. *Trends in Endocrinological Metabolism*. 13: 75–78.; c) Zamzami, N., et al. (1996) Mitochondrial control of nuclear apoptosis. *Journal of Experimental Medicine*. 183: 1533-1544.

9. Smith, Ryan (2007) Study shows DCA suppresses cancer without damaging normal cells. *Folio University of Alberta*. 44 (11), February 2.

10. Koch, W. F. (1961) *The Survival Factor in Neoplastic and Viral Disease: An Introduction to Carbonyl and Free Radical Therapy*. Detroit, MI: Vanderkloot Press.

11. http://www.chironclinic.com/article-winning_the_war_on_cancer.html.

12. Fahey, J. W., et al. (1997) Broccoli sprouts: An exceptionally rich source of inducers of enzymes that protect against chemical carcinogens. *Proceedings of the National Academy of Sciences*. 94: 10367-10372.

13. Seyfried, Thomas (2012) *Cancer as a Metabolic Disease: On the Origin, Management, and Prevention of Cancer*. New York: Wiley & Son.

14. Dongjun, W., et al. (2014) Cell state-specific metabolic dependency in hematopoiesis and leukemogenesis. *Cell*. 158 (6): 1309–1323.

15. Magee, B. A., et al. (1979) The inhibition of malignant cell growth by ketone bodies. *Australian Journal of Experimental Biology and Medical Science*. 57 (5): 529-39.

16. Schmidt, M., et al. (2011) Effects of a ketogenic diet on the quality of life in 16 patients with advanced cancer: A pilot trial. *Nutritional Metabolism (London)*. 8 (1): 54.

17. a) Fine, Eugene J. (2012) Targeting insulin inhibition as a metabolic therapy in advanced cancer: A pilot safety and feasibility dietary trial in 10 patients. *Nutrition*. 28: 1028-1035; b) Abdelwahab, Mohammed G., et al. (2012)

The Ketogenic Diet Is an Effective Adjuvant to Radiation Therapy for the Treatment of Malignant Glioma. *PLoS ONE.* 7 (5): e36197 DOI.

18. Ho., Victor W., et al. (2011) A Low Carbohydrate, High Protein Diet Slows Tumor Growth and Prevents Cancer Initiation. *Cancer Research.* 71 (13): 4484–93.

19. Eugene J. Fine, et al. (2012) Targeting insulin inhibition as a metabolic therapy in advanced cancer: A pilot safety and feasibility dietary trial in 10 patients. *Nutrition.* 28 (10): 1028-1035.

20. Johnson, Lorie (2013) Starving Cancer: Ketogenic Diet a Key to Recovery. *CBN News Medical Reporter.* Friday, June 21.

21. a) Poff, A. M., et al. (2013) The Ketogenic Diet and Hyperbaric Oxygen Therapy Prolong Survival in Mice with Systemic Metastatic Cancer. *PLoS ONE* 8 (6): e65522. doi:10.1371/journal.pone.0065522; b) Poff, A. M., et al. (2014) Ketone Supplementation Decreases Tumor Cell Viability and Prolongs Survival of Mice with Metastatic Cancer. *International Journal of Cancer.* 44 (6), 1843-52.

22. Bowden, Jonny & Sinatra, Stephen (2012) *The Great Cholesterol Myth: Why Lowering Your Cholesterol Won't Prevent Heart Disease-and the Statin-Free Plan That Will.* Fair Winds Press.

23. Westman, Eric C. & Moore, Jimmy (2013) *Cholesterol Clarity.* North Clarendon, VT: Tuttle Publishing.

24. Seyfried, Thomas N., et al. (2014) Cancer as a Metabolic Disease: Implications for Novel Therapeutics. *Carcinogenesis.* 35: 515–27.

25. Schernhammer, E. S., et al. (2012) Consumption of artificial sweetener–and sugar-containing soda and risk of lymphoma and leukemia in men and women. *American Journal of Clinical Nutrition.* 96: 1419–28.

26. a) Fuhrman, Joel (2003) *Eat for Health.* New York: Little Brown & Company; b) Fuhrman, Joel (2011) *Super Immunity: The Essential Nutrition Guide for Boosting Your Body's Defenses to Live Longer, Stronger, and Disease Free.* New York: HarperOne.

27. Ingram, D. (1994) Diet and Subsequent Survival in Women with Breast Cancer. *British Journal of Cancer.* 69 (3): 592-595.

28. a) Chan, J. M., et al. (2006) Diet after Diagnosis and the Risk of Prostate Progression, Recurrence, and Death. *Cancer Causes and Control.* 17 (2): 199-208; b) Canene-Adams, et al. (2007) Combinations of Tomato and Broccoli Enhance Anti-Tumor Activity in Dunning R3327-H Prostate Adenocarcinomas. *Cancer Research.* 67 (2): 836-43; c) Wagner, A. E., et al. (2013) Health Promoting Effects of Brassica-derived Phytochemicals. *Oxidative Medicine and Cellular Longevity.* 2013: 964539; d) Gerhauser, C. (2013) Epigenetic Impact of Dietary

Isothiocyanates in Cancer Chemoprevention. *Current Opinion in Clinical Nutrition and Metabolic Care.* 16 (4): 405-10.

29. Eccles, Nyjon (2013) *Winning the War on Cancer.* The Chiron Clinic, London. http://www.chironclinic.com/article-winning_the_war_on_cancer .html.

30. *University of Southampton Press Release* July 9, 2013: Scientists develop ground-breaking new method of 'starving' cancer cells. Ref: 13/129.

31. Leprivier, Gabriel, et al. (2013) The eEF2 Kinase Confers Resistance to Nutrient Deprivation by Blocking Translation Elongation. *Cell.* DOI: 10.1016/j.cell.2013.04.055.

32. Koch, W. F. (1961) *The Survival Factor in Neoplastic and Viral Disease.* Detroit, MI: Vanderkloot Press.

33. Haley, Daniel (2000) *Politics in Healing: Suppression and Manipulation of American Medicine.* Washington, DC: Potomac Valley Press.

34. Szent-Gyorgi, A., et al. (1963) Cancer Therapy: A Possible New Approach. *Science.* 140: 1391-1392.

35. http://www.angio.org/

36. http://www.healncure.com/can-we-eat-to-starve-cancer/

37. a) Lockwood, K. (1994) Partial and complete regression of breast cancer in patients in relation to dosage of coenzyme Q10. *Biochemical and Biophysical Research Communications.* 199 (3): 1504-8; b) Lockwood, K., et al. (1995) Progress on therapy of breast cancer with coenzyme Q10 and the regression of metastases. *Biochemical and Biophysical Research Communications.* 212 (1): 172-7.

38. Folkers, K., et al. (1997) Activities of coenzyme Q10 in animal models and a serious deficiency in patients with cancer. *Biochemical and Biophysical Research Communications.* 234 (2): 296-9)

39. Hodges, S., et al. (1999) CoQ10: could it have a role in cancer management? *Biofactors.* 9 (2-4): 365-370.

40. Dreher, D. L. & Junod, A. F. (1996) Role of oxygen free radicals in cancer development. *European Journal of Cancer.* 32A (1): 30-8.

41. a) Giugliano, Dario, et al. (2008) Glucose metabolism and hyperglycemia. *American Journal of Clinical Nutrition.* 87 (1) 217S-222S; b) Ceriello, A. (2006) Oxidative stress and diabetes-associated complications. *Endocrine Practice* 12 Supplement. 1: 60-62.

42. a) Wang, Jie & Yi, Jing (2008) Cancer cell killing via ROS: To increase or decrease, that is the question. *Cancer Biology and Therapy.* 7 (12): 1875-1884; b) Nogueira, Veronique & Hay, Nissim (2013) Molecular Pathways: Reactive Oxygen Species Homeostasis in Cancer Cells and Implications for Cancer Therapy. *Clinical Cancer Research;* 19 (16): 4309–14.

43. Goggins, Alden & Matten, Glen (2012) *The Health Delusion: How to Achieve Exceptional Health in the 21ˢᵗ Century.* London: Hay House.

44. Goepp, Julius (2008) Coenzyme Q10 and Cancer Enhancing Treatment Outcomes and Improving Chemotherapy Tolerability. *Life Extension Magazine.* February.

45. a) Kaiser, Jocelyn (2014) Antioxidants Could Spur Tumors by Acting on Cancer Gene. *Science.* 343: 477; b) Bouayed, J. & Bohn, T. (2010) *Oxidative Medicine and Cellular Longevity.* 3 (4): 228-237.

46. Bjelakovic, G., et al. (2012) Antioxidant supplements for prevention of mortality in healthy participants and patients with various diseases. Published Online: Cochrane Summaries. March 14.

47. http://www.wellnessresources.com/health/articles/ubiquinol_q10_anti-aging_properties/.

48. Hoffman, Jay M. (1996) *Hunza: Secrets of the World's Healthiest and Oldest Living People.* El Monte, CA: New Win Publishing.

49. Taylor, Renée (1964). *Long Suppressed Hunza Health Secrets for Long Life and Happiness.* New York: Award Books.

50. Milazzo, Stefania, et al. (2011). Laetrile treatment for cancer. In Milazzo, Stefania. *Cochrane Database of Systematic Reviews.* doi:10.1002/14651858. CD005476.pub3.

51. a) Chen, Liu Qi, et al. (2013) Evaluations of extracellular pH within in vivo tumors using acidoCEST MRI. *Magnetic Resonance in Medicine.* 26 NOV, DOI: 10.1002/mrm.25053; b) Robey, Ian F., et al. (2009) Bicarbonate Increases Tumor pH and Inhibits Spontaneous Metastases. *Cancer Research.* 69: (6) 2260-2268; c) https://camel.arizona.edu/cancer_and_baking_soda.

52. (a) Li, X., et al. (2013) Traditional Chinese medicine in cancer care: a review of controlled clinical studies published in Chinese. *PLoS One.* 8. (4): e60338; b) Liu, J., et al. (2011) Traditional Chinese medicine in cancer care: a review of case reports published in Chinese literature. *Forsch Komplementmedizin.* 18 (5): 257-63; and c) Yang, Gong, et al. (2012) Traditional Chinese medicine in cancer care: a review of case series published in the Chinese literature. *Journal of Evidence-Based Complementary Alternative Medicine.* Volume 2012: Article ID 751046.

53. Yang, Gong, et al. (2013) Prediagnosis Soy Food Consumption and Lung Cancer Survival in Women. *Journal of Clinical Oncology.* 2013: 1548-1553.

54. Lai, Henry C., et al. (2013) Development of artemisinin compounds for cancer treatment. *Investigational New Drugs.* 31: 230–246.

55. Moen, I. & Stuhr, L. E. (2012) Hyperbaric oxygen therapy and cancer—a review. *Targeted Oncology.* 7 (4): 233-42.

56. a) http://cellfood-atm.blogspot.com/; b) Nuvoli, Barbara, et al. (2014) CELLFOOD™ induces apoptosis in human mesothelioma and colorectal cancer cells by modulating p53, c-myc and pAkt signaling pathways. *Journal of Experimental & Clinical Cancer Research.* 33: 24 doi:10.1186/1756-9966-33-24; c) Catalani, S., et al (2013) Metabolism modifications and apoptosis induction after Cellfood administration to leukemia cell lines. *Journal of Experimental and Clinical Cancer Research.* 32: 63.

57. a) Ornish, Dean, et al. (2008) Changes in prostate gene expression in men undergoing an intensive nutrition and lifestyle intervention. *Proceedings of the National Academy of Sciences.* 105 (24): 8369-8374; b) Frattaroli, J., et al. (2008) Clinical events in prostate cancer lifestyle trial: results from two years of follow-up. *Urology.* 72 (6): 1319-23; c) Ornish, D., et al. (2013) Effect of comprehensive lifestyle changes on telomerase activity and telomere length in men with biopsy-proven low-risk prostate cancer: 5-year follow-up of a descriptive pilot study. *Lancet Oncology.* 14 (11):1112-20.

58. Richmond, C., et al. (2007) Societal Resources and Thriving Health: A New Approach for Understanding the Health of Indigenous Canadians. *American Journal of Public Health.* 97 (10) 1827-1833.

59. a) Gago-Dominguez, M. J., et al. (2003) Opposing Effects of Dietary n-3 and n-6 Acids on Mammary Carcinogenesis. *British Journal of Cancer.* 89 (9) 1686-92; b) Goodstine, S. L., et al. (2003) Dietary Fatty Acid Ratio: Possible Relationship to Premenopausal but Not Postmenopausal Breast Cancer Risk in U.S. Women. *Journal of Nutrition.* 133 (5) 1409-14; c) Leitzmann, M. M., et al. (2004) Dietary Intake of n-3 and n-6 Fatty Acids and the Risk of Prostate Cancer. *American Journal of Clinical Nutrition.* 80: 204-216; d) Norat, T. S., et al (2005) Meat, Fish and Colorectal Cancer Risk. *Journal of the National Cancer Institute.* 97 (12) 906-916; e) Terry, P. A., et al (2002) Fatty Fish Lowers the Risk of Endometrial Cancer. *Cancer Epidemiology, Biomarkers and Prevention.* 11 (1): 143-145; f) Terry, P. A., et al. (2001) Fatty Fish Consumption and Risk of Prostate Cancer. *Lancet.* 357 (9270): 1764-66.

Chapter Eleven - What You Can Do Now to Complement Your Cancer Treatment

1. Singh, Shinjini, et al. (2015) Genome-Based Multitargeting of Cancer: Hype or Hope? In Aggarwal, et al. (Eds.) *Multitargeted Approach to Treatment of Cancer.* Heidelberg, Germany: Springer Production.

2. Servan-Schreiber, David (2009) *Anticancer: A New Way of Life.* New York: Viking.

3. Chang, Raymond (2012) *Beyond the Magic Bullet: The Anti-cancer Cocktail.* Garden City Park, NY: Square One Publishers.

4. a) http://www.ketogenic-diet-resource.com/cancer-treatments.html; b) Woolf, Eric C. & Scheck, Adrienne C. (2012) Metabolism and glioma therapy. *CNS Oncology.* 1 (1): 7–10.

5. a) Safdie, Fernando M. (2009) Fasting and Cancer Treatment in Humans: A Case series report. *Aging.* 1 (12): 988–1007; b) Fine, Eugene J., et al. (2012) Targeting insulin inhibition as a metabolic therapy in advanced cancer: A pilot safety and feasibility dietary trial in 10 patients. *Nutrition.* 28: 1028–1035; c) Klement, Rainer J. & Champ, Colin E. (2014) Calories, carbohydrates, and cancer therapy with radiation: exploiting the five R's through dietary manipulation. *Cancer Metastasis Review.* 33: 217–229.

6. Kamiński, S. (2007) Polymorphism of bovine beta-casein and its potential effect on human health. *Journal of Applied Genetics.* 48 (3): 189-98.

7. a) Dowling, Ryan J. O., et al. (2011) Understanding the benefit of metformin use in cancer treatment. *BMC Medicine.* 9: 33. b) http://www.webmd.com/cancer/news/20121130/diabetes-drug-metformin-cancer.

8. http://www.cancer.gov/cancertopics/research-updates/2013/metformin.

9. Perlmutter, David (2013) *Grain Brain: The Surprising Truth about Wheat, Carbs, and Sugar-Your Brain's Silent Killers.* New York: Little, Brown & Company.

10. a) Zhang, Chi, et al. (2014) Cancer may be a pathway to cell survival under persistent hypoxia and elevated ROS: A model for solid-cancer initiation and early development. *International Journal of Cancer.* Published online: 27 May; b) Somlyai, Gábor (2002) *Defeating Cancer! The Biological Effect of Deuterium Depletion.* London: AuthorHouse; c) Gyöngyi, Z., et al. (2013) Deuterium depleted water effects on survival of lung cancer patients and expression of Kras, Bcl2, and Myc genes in mouse lung. *Nutrition and Cancer.* 65 (2): 240-246.

11. a) http://cellfood-atm.blogspot.com/; b) Nuvoli, Barbara, et al. (2014) CELLFOOD™ induces apoptosis in human mesothelioma and colorectal cancer cells by modulating p53, c-myc and pAkt signaling pathways. *Journal of Experimental & Clinical Cancer Research.* 33 (1) 24; c) Catalani, S., et al. (2013) Metabolism modifications and apoptosis induction after Cellfood administration to leukemia cell lines. *Journal of Experimental and Clinical Cancer Research.* 32: 63.

12. http://www.amazon.com/Cellfood-Liquid-Concentrate-1-Ounce-Bottle/dp/B000F4F9JS

13. a) http://www.canceractive.com/cancer-active-page-link.aspx?n=3132; b) Tomaselli, F., et al. (2001) Acute effects of combined photodynamic therapy and hyperbaric oxygenation in lung cancer. *Lasers in Surgery and Medicine.* 28 (5): 399-403; c) Maier, A., et al. (2000) Combined photodynamic therapy and

hyperbaric oxygenation in carcinoma of the esophagus and the esophago-gastric junction. *European Journal of Cardiothoracic Surgery.* 18 (6): 649-54; d) Chen, Q., et al. (2002) Improvement of tumor response by manipulation of tumor oxygenation during photodynamic therapy. *Journal of Photochemistry and Photobiology.* 76 (2): 197-203.

14. a) World Health Organization, GLOBOCAN, 2008 data; b) http://www.worldlifeexpectancy.com/cause-of-death/all-cancers/by-country/; c) Sinha, R., et al. (2003) Cancer Risk and Diet in India. *Journal of Postgraduate Medicine.* 49: 222-228.

15. a) Anand, Preetha, et al. (2008) Curcumin and cancer: An "old-age" disease with an "age-old" solution. *Cancer Letters.* 267: 133–164; b) Hasima, Noor & Aggarwal, Bharat B. (2012) Cancer-linked targets modulated by curcumin. *International Journal of Biochemistry and Molecular Biology.* 3 (4): 328-351; c) Hasima, Noor & Aggarwal, Bharat B. (2014) Targeting Proteasomal Pathways by Dietary Curcumin for Cancer Prevention and Treatment. *Current Medicinal Chemistry.* 21; d) Ravindran, Jayaraj, et al. (2009) Curcumin and Cancer Cells: How Many Ways Can Curry Kill Tumor Cells Selectively? *American Association of Pharmaceutical Scientists Journal.* 11 (3): 495–510; e) Aggarwal, Bharat B. (2014) Molecular Targets and Therapeutic Use of Curcumin. 3rd *Annual Conference and Expo IV Therapies 2014 Integrative Oncology,* January 25; f) Anand, Preetha, et al. (2008) Curcumin and cancer: An "old-age" disease with an "age-old" solution. *Cancer Letters.* 267: 133–164; g) Hasima, Noor & Aggarwal, Bharat B. (2012) Cancer-linked targets modulated by curcumin. *International Journal of Biochemistry and Molecular Biology.* 3 (4): 328-351; h) Hasima, Noor & Aggarwal, Bharat B. (2014) Targeting Proteasomal Pathways by Dietary Curcumin for Cancer Prevention and Treatment. *Current Medicinal Chemistry.* 21; i) Ravindran, Jayaraj, et al. (2009) Curcumin and Cancer Cells: How Many Ways Can Curry Kill Tumor Cells Selectively? *American Association of Pharmaceutical Scientists Journal.* 11 (3): 495–510; j) Bharti, Alok C., et al. (2003) Curcumin Inhibits Constitutive and Interleukin-6-Inducible STAT3 Phosphorylation in Human Multiple Myeloma Cells. *Journal of Immunology.* 171 (7): 3863; k) Aggarwal, Bharat B. (2014) Molecular Targets and Therapeutic Use of Curcumin. 3rd *Annual Conference and Expo IV Therapies 2014 Integrative Oncology,* January 25; l) Shehzad, A., Wahid F. & Lee Y. S. (2010) Curcumin in cancer chemoprevention: molecular targets, pharmacokinetics, bioavailability, and clinical trials. *Archives of Pharmacology (Weinheim).* 343 (9): 489-99; m) Johnson, J. J. & Mukhtar, H. (2007) Curcumin for chemoprevention of colon cancer. *Cancer Letters.* 255 (2):170-81.

16. Goel, A. & Aggarwal, B. B. (2010) Curcumin, the golden spice from Indian saffron, is a chemosensitizer and radiosensitizer for tumors and chemoprotector and radioprotector for normal organs. *Nutrition and Cancer.* 62 (7): 919-30.

17. a) http://umm.edu/health/medical/altmed/herb/turmeric#ixzz33K2jt8Ld; b) http://www.ragtaghealth.com/products/view/turmeric.

18. http://ahccresearch.com/.

19. a) http://www.cancer.gov/cancertopics/pdq/cam/milkthistle/Patient/page2; b) Manna, Sunil K., et al. (1999) Silymarin Suppresses TNF-Induced Activation of NF-kB, c-JunN-Terminal Kinase, and Apoptosis1.*The Journal of Immunology.* 163: 6800–6809; c) Ramasamy, Kumaraguruparan & Agarwal, Rajesh (2008) Multitargeted therapy of cancer by silymarin. *Cancer Letters.* 269 (2): 352–362.

20. Holmes, Michelle, D., et al. (2010) Aspirin Intake and Survival after Breast Cancer. *Journal of Clinical Oncology.* 28: 1467-1472.

21. (a) Garland, Cedric F., et al. (2011) Vitamin D Supplement Doses and Serum 25-Hydroxyvitamin D in the Range Associated with Cancer Prevention. *Anticancer Research.* 31: 617-622; b) Gandini, S., et al. (2011) Meta-analysis of observational studies of serum 25-hydroxyvitamin D levels and colorectal, breast and prostate cancer and colorectal adenoma. *International Journal of Cancer.* 128: 1414-1424; c) Moukayed, M. & Grant, W. B. (2013) Molecular link between vitamin D and cancer prevention. *Nutrients.* 5: 3993-4021; Bjelakovic, G., et al. (2014) Vitamin D supplementation for prevention of mortality in adults. *Cochrane Database Systematic Reviews.* 1: CD007470.

22. http://www.healthy-lifestyle-store.com/terramin-edible-clay-5.

23. a) Gaynor, Mitchell (2002) *The Healing Power of Sound: Recovery from Life-Threatening Illness Using Sound, Voice, and Music.* Boston, MA: Shambhala Publications; b) www.gaynoroncology.com; c) http://www.omcrystalsinging-bowls.com/.

24. Grassi, Luigi & Riba, Michelle (Eds.) (2014) *Psychopharmacology and Palliative Care.* New York: Springer.

25. http://www.webmd.com/cancer/features/exercise-cancer-patients.

26. Grassi, Luigi & Riba, Michelle (2012) *Clinical Psycho-oncology: An International Perspective.* New York: Wiley-Blackwell.

27. a) http://fivetothriveplan.com/; b) Alschuler, Lise & Gazella, Karolyn A. (2013) *The Definitive Guide to Thriving After Cancer: A Five-Step Integrative Plan to Reduce the Risk of Recurrence and Build Lifelong Health.* New York: Ten Speed Press.

Chapter Twelve - Taking Charge of Being
a Care Recipient or a Caregiver

1. Fraser Health (2005) *Handbook for Caregivers*. Vancouver, British Columbia, Canada.

2. a) Kübler-Ross, Elizabeth (1969) *On Death and Dying*. New York: Routledge; b) Kübler-Ross, Elizabeth (2005) *On Grief and Grieving: Finding the Meaning of Grief Through the Five Stages of Loss*. New York: Simon & Schuster.

3. a) http://familydoctor.org/familydoctor/en/healthcare-management/end-of-life-issues/; b) http://hospicenet.org/.

4. National Cancer Institute. When Someone You Love Has Advanced Cancer: Support for Caregivers. http://www.cancer.gov/. American Cancer Society: http://www.cancer.org/treatment/caregivers/caregiving/index

5. Dehaene, Stanislas (2014) *Consciousnesss and the Brain: Deciphering How the Brain Codes Our Thoughts*. New York: Viking.

6. Westman, Jack C. (1997) *Born to Belong: Becoming Who I Am*. Lima, OH: CSS Publishing Company.

7. Rohr, Richard (2013) *Immortal Diamond*. New York: Jossey-Bass, p. 23.

8. Kabat-Zinn, Jon (2013) *Full Catastrophe Living (Revised Edition): Using the Wisdom of Your Body and Mind to Face Stress, Pain, and Illness*. New York: Bantam Books.

9. Lutz, A., et al. (2004) Long-term meditators self-induce high-amplitude gamma synchrony during mental practice. *Proceedings of the National Academy of Sciences*. 101: 16369-73.

10. Pickert, Kate (2014) The Art of Being Mindful. *Time*. February 3, pp. 41-46.

11. Ibid.

12. Teno, Joan M., et al. (2013) Change in End-of-Life Care for Medicare Beneficiaries: Site of Death, Place of Care, and Health Care Transitions in 2000, 2005, and 2009. *Journal of the American Medical Association*. 309 (5): 470-477.

13. http://www.dartmouthatlas.org/.

14. Christakis, Nicholas A. (1999) *Death Foretold: Prophecy and Prognosis in Medical Care*. Chicago, Ill.: University of Chicago Press.

15. Gorenstein, Dan (2013) How Doctors Die: Showing Others the Way. *The New York Times*. November 19, p. F1.

16. a) Byock, Ira (1998) *Dying Well*. New York: Putnam/RiverHead; b) Byock, Ira (2013) *The Best Possible Care*. New York: Avery Books/Penguin; c) http://www.dyingwell.org; d) http://www.dyingwell.org/discguide.htm.

17. Dolan, Susan R. & Vizzard, Audrey (2013) *The End of Life Advisor: Personal, Legal, and Medical Considerations for a Peaceful, Dignified Death*. Denver, CO: Outskirts Press.

18. Brody, Jane (2009) *Guide to Great Beyond*. New York: Random House.

19. a) Pausch, Randy with Zaslow, Jeffrey (2008) *The Last Lecture*. Hyperion; b) www.cmu.edu/uls/journeys/randy-pausch.

20. op. cit. Gorenstein.

21. Nuland, Sherwin B. (1995) *How We Die, Reflections on Life's Final Chapter*. New York: Vintage Books. Study Guide & Plot Summary http://www.bookrags.com/studyguide-how-we-die/ BookRags and Gale's For Students Series.

22. Gubar, Susan (2013) Living With Cancer: Giving Thanks and Latkes. *The New York Times*. November 27.

23. http://www.webmd.com/parenting/helping-children-who-are-grieving#.

24. http://www.teachersandfamilies.com/open/parent/grief5.cfm.

25. http://www.CompassionAndChoices.org.

26. Tillich, Paul (1948) *The Shaking of the Foundations*. New York: C. Scribner's Sons.

27. Manning, Douglas (2011) *Don't Take My Grief Away from Me*. Oklahoma City, OK: In-Sight Books, Inc.

28. Siegel, Bernie (2009) *Faith, Hope and Healing: Inspiring Lessons Learned from People Living with Cancer*. Nashville, TN: Turner Publishing Company.

29. Servan-Schreiber, David (2009) *Anticancer: A New Way of Life*. New York: Viking.

Chapter Thirteen - Where Are We Now?

1. Link, Michael P. (2013) Collaborating to Conquer Cancer: Lessons From Our Children. *Journal of Clinical Oncology*. 31 (7): 825-832.

2. Centers for Disease Control and Prevention (2011). Cancer survivors—United States, 2007. *Morbidity and Mortality Weekly Report*. 60 (9): 269–272.

3. Leaf, Clifton (2013) *The Truth in Small Doses: Why We're Losing the War on Cancer-and How to Win It*. New York: Simon and Schuster.

4. Pollack, Andrew (2013) Promising New Cancer Drugs Empower the Body's Own Defense System. *The New York Times*. June 3, 2013.

5. Editorial (2013) The failure of cancer medicine? *The Lancet*. 381 (9865): 423.

6. Akst, Jef (2014) The Dark Side of Curing Cancer: Panelists at AACR discuss the health risks that cancer survivors must face. *The Scientist*. April 7.

7.   http://fundedresearch.cancer.gov/.

8.   Ryan Gilbert, Budget Analyst of National Cancer Institute; 301-435-2607; ryan.gilbert@nih.gov.

9.   *Cancer-Changing The Conversation: The Nation's Investment In Cancer Research: An annual plan and budget proposal for fiscal year 2012.* Washington, DC: National Cancer Institute.

10. a) Varmus, Harold & Harlow, Ed (2012) Science funding: Provocative questions in cancer research. *Nature.* 481: 436-437; b) http://provocativequestions. nci.nih.gov/.

11. Office of Budget and Finance (2013) *Plan and Budget Proposal.* Washington, DC: National Cancer Institute.

12. Willoughby, Jack (2013) The New Science Behind Medical Investing. *Barron's.* October 21, pp. 44-45.

Chapter Fourteen - Obstacles to Progress

1.   Link, Michael P. (2013) Collaborating to Conquer Cancer: Lessons From Our Children. *Journal of Clinical Oncology.* 31 (7): 825-832.

2.   Brawley, Otis W. with Goldberg, Paul (2012) *How We Do Harm: A Doctor Breaks Ranks About Being Sick in America.* New York: St. Martin's Griffin.

3.   Proctor, Robert N. (1995) *Cancer Wars: How Politics Shapes What We Know and Don't Know about Cancer.* New York: Basic Books.

4.   Davis, Devra (2007) *The Secret History of the War on Cancer.* New York: Basic Books.

5.   Epstein, Samuel S. (2005) *Cancer-gate: How to Win the Losing Cancer War.* Amityville, NY: Baywood Publishing Company.

6.   Hartocollis, Anemona (2013) Cancer Centers Racing to Map Patients' Genes. *New York Times.* April 21, p. A1.

7.   Pear, Robert (2013) Doctors Who Profit From Radiation Prescribe It More Often, Study Finds. *The New York Times,* August 18.

8.   Griffin, G. Edward (1997) *World Without Cancer. Second Edition.* American Media.

9.   Abramson, John D. (2004) *Overdosed America: The Broken Promise of American Medicine.* New York: HarperCollins.

10. Abramson, John D. & Redberg, Rita F. (2013) Don't Give More Patients Statins. *The New York Times.* November 14, p. A27.

11. Welch, H. Gilbert, Schwartz, Lisa M., & Woloshin, Steven (2011) *Overdiagnosed: Making People Sick in the Pursuit of Health*. Boston, MA: Beacon Press.

12. a) http://www.cancer.gov/cancertopics/cam; b) Horneber, M., et al. (2012) How many cancer patients use complementary and alternative medicine: a systematic review and meta-analysis. *Integrative Cancer Therapies*. 11 (3): 187-203.)

13. Offit, Paul (2013) *Do You Believe in Magic? The Sense and Nonsense of Alternative Medicine*. New York: Harper.

14. Salzberg, Steven (2013) Alternative Medicine Providers Show Their Greedy Side. *Forbes*. August 26.

15. Goldhill, David (2013) *Catastrophic Care: How American Health Care Killed My Father—And How We Can Fix It*. New York: Knopf.

16. a) https://osf.io/ezcuj/wiki/home/; b)http://centerforopenscience.org/.

17. a) Rehman, Jalees (2013) Cancer research in crisis: Are the drugs we count on based on bad science? *Salon*. Sep 1, 2013; b) Begley, C., et al. (2012) Drug development: Raise standards for preclinical cancer research. *Nature*. 483: 531–533.

18. Mobley, Aaron, et al. (2013) A Survey on Data Reproducibility in Cancer Research Provides Insights into Our Limited Ability to Translate Findings from the Laboratory to the Clinic. *Plos One*. May 15.

19. Orenstein, Peggy (2013) The Problem with Pink: Our Feel-Good War on Breast Cancer. *The New York Times Magazine*. April 28, pp. 37-71.

20. Bleyer, Archie & Welch, H. Gilbert (2012) Effect of Three Decades of Screening Mammography on Breast-Cancer Incidence. *New England Journal of Medicine*. 367: 1998-2005.

21. Orenstein, Peggy (2013) The Problem with Pink: Our Feel-Good War on Breast Cancer. *The New York Times Magazine*. April 28, pp. 37-71.

22. King, Samantha (2006) *PINK RIBBONS, INC.: Breast Cancer and the Politics of Philanthropy*. Minneapolis: University of Minnesota Press.

23. Palmer, Chris (2013) Q&A: The Cancer Tradeoff. Physicist-turned-oncologist Robert Austin argues that cancer is a natural consequence of our rapid evolution. *The Scientist*. April 3.

24. Johnson, George (2013) *The Cancer Chronicles: Unlocking Medicine's Deepest Mystery*. New York: Knopf.

25. Marks, Paul & Sterngold, James (2014) *On the Cancer Frontier: One Man, One Disease, and a Medical Revolution*. New York: Public Affairs

26. The Editorial Board (2013) Another Alleged Drug Kickback Scheme. *The New York Times*. April 24.

27. Goldacre, Ben (2013) *Bad Pharma: How Drug Companies Mislead Companies and Harm Patients*. New York: Faber & Faber.

Chapter Fifteen - Where Do We Go from Here?

1. Cancer Medicine (2013) Withdrawing treatment makes some cancers stop growing. *The Economist*. April 13, p. 81.

2. Link, Michael P. (2013) Collaborating to Conquer Cancer: Lessons from Our Childen. *Journal of Clinical Oncology*. 31 (7): 825-828.

3. Cancer-Changing The Conversation: The Nation's Investment In Cancer Research: An annual plan and budget proposal for fiscal year 2012. Washington, DC: National Cancer Institute.

4. a) Balogh, Erin, Patlak, Margie & Nass, Sharyl J. (2013) *Delivering Affordable Cancer Care in the 21ˢᵗ Century: Workshop Summary*. Institute of Medicine, National Academy of Sciences: National Academies Press; b) Levit, Laura (2013) *Delivering High-Quality Cancer Care: Charting a New Course for a System in Crisis*. Washington, DC: The National Academies Press.

5. Saporito, Bill with Park, Alice (2013) The Conspiracy To End Cancer. *Time*. April 1.

6. Saulnier, Beth (2014) Bench to Bedside. *Cornell Alumni Magazine*. May-June, pp. 53-57.

7. op. cit. Saparito

8. http://www.cancer.gov/cancertopics/tobacco/smoking/.

9. a) http://www.cancer.org/cancer/cancercauses/dietandphysicalactivity/body-weightandcancerrisk/body-weight-and-cancer-risk-effects; b) http://www.cancer.gov/cancertopics/factsheet/Risk/obesity.

10. Federico, Alessandro, et al. (2010) Fat: A matter of disturbance for the immune system. *World Journal of Gastroenterology*. 16 (38): 4762–4772.

11. Kaiser, Jocelyn (2013) Cholesterol Forges Link Between Obesity and Breast Cancer. *Science*. 342: 1028.

12. Ropiek, David (2013) Taming Radiation Fears. *The New York Times*. October 22, p. A21.

13. Yablokov, Alexey, Nesterenko, Alexey, & Nesterenko, Vassili (2009) *Chernobyl: Consequences of the Catastrophe for People and the Environment*. New York: New York Academy of Sciences.

14. http://www.lungcancertrusts.com/.

15. http://www.scientificamerican.com/article/cancer-the-march-on-malignancy/ Volume 311, No. 1.

16. a) Brody, Julia Green, et al. (2014) Breast Cancer and Environmental Research. *Science*. 344 (6184): 577; b) President's Cancer Panel (2010) Reducing environmental cancer risk: What we can do now. Washington, DC. U.S. Department

of Health and Human Services, National Institutes of Health, National Cancer Institute.

17. Division of Environmental Health Assessment Center for Environmental Health (2008) Love Canal Follow-up Health Study. Albany, NY: State of New York Department of Health.

18. Bove, Frank J., et al. (2014) Evaluation of mortality among marines and navy personnel exposed to contaminated drinking water at USMC base camp Lejeune: a retrospective cohort study. *Environmental Health.* 13: 10 doi:10.1186/1476-069X-13-10.

19. http://www.brockovich.com/.

20. http://www.cdc.gov/nceh/clusters/about.htm.

21. a) American Chemical Society (2008) Lead Leaching and Faucet Corrosion In PVC Home Plumbing. *ScienceDaily.* Retrieved December 22; b) Miranda, Marie Lynn, et al. (2007). "Changes in Blood Lead Levels Associated with Use of Chloramines in Water Treatment Systems". *Environmental Health Perspectives.* 115 (2): 221–5.

22. Zhang, et al. (2008) Nitrification in Premise Plumbing: Role of Phosphate, pH and Pipe Corrosion. *Environmental Science & Technology.* 42 (12): 4280-4.

23. http://www.medicinenet.com/plastic/page3.htm.

24. Richardson, Ruth E., et al. (2011) Investigation of factors affecting the accumulation of vinyl chloride in polyvinyl chloride piping used in drinking water distribution systems. *Water Research.* 45 (8): 2607–2615.

25. http://www.euractiv.com/specialreport-plastics-pvc/pvc-industry-sees-looming-clash-news-516437 07 December 2012.

26. National Research Council (2006) *Health Risks from Exposure to Low Levels of Ionizing Radiation: BEIR VII Phase 2.* Washington, DC: The National Academies Press.

27. Berrington de González, A., et al. (2009) Projected cancer risks from computed tomographic scans performed in the United States in 2007. *Archives of Internal Medicine.* 169 (22): 2071-7.

28. Smith-Bindman, R. (2012) Environmental causes of breast cancer and radiation from medical imaging: findings from the Institute of Medicine report. *Archives of Internal Medicine.* 172 (13): 1023-7.

29. Redberg, Rita F. & Smith-Bindman, Rebecca (2014) We Are Giving Ourselves Cancer. *The New York Times.* January 31, p. A21.

30. Storrs, Carina (2013) How Much Do CT Scans Increase the Risk of Cancer? *Scientific American.* July, p. 32.

31. Reuben, Suzzane H. (2010) *Reducing Environmental Cancer Risk: What We Can Do Now.* Washington, DC: National Cancer Institute.

32. http://www.cancer.gov/cancertopics/factsheet/Risk/cellphones.

33. Prostate Cancer: Help or Harm. *The Economist*. March 8, 2014, pp. 85-86.

34. Leary, Rebecca J., et al. (2012) Detection of Chromosomal Alterations in the Circulation of Cancer Patients with Whole-Genome Sequencing. *Science Translational Medicine*. 4 (162): 162ra154.

35. a) Banki, Farzaneh, et al. (2007) Plasma DNA as a Molecular Marker for Completeness of Resection and Recurrent Disease in Patients with Esophageal Cancer. *Archives of Surgery*. 142: 533-539; b) Ghorbian, S. & Ardekani, Ali M. (2012) Non-Invasive Detection of Esophageal Cancer using Genetic Changes in Circulating Cell-Free DNA. *Avicenna Journal of Medical Biotechnology*. 4 (1): 3-13; c) Shaw, J. A., et al. (2011) Circulating tumor cells and plasma DNA analysis in patients with indeterminate early or metastatic breast cancer. *Biomarkers in Medicine*. 5 (1): 87-91.

36. http://www.sri.com.

37. Morré, James & Morré, Dorothy (2013) *ECTO-NOX Proteins*. New York: Springer. www.oncoblotlabs.com.

38. Diehl, Frank, et al. (2008) Circulating mutant DNA to assess tumor dynamics. *Nature Medicine*. 14 (9): 985-990.

39. Aćimović, Srdjan S., et al. (2014) LSPR Chip for Parallel, Rapid, and Sensitive Detection of Cancer Markers in Serum. *Nano Letters*. 14 (5): 2636 DOI: 10.1021/nl500574n.

40. Imperiale, Thomas F., et al. (2014) Multitarget Stool DNA Testing for Colorectal-Cancer Screening. *New England Journal of Medicine*. 370: 1287-1297.

41. http://metabolomx.com/2012/10/23/biocentury-feature-sniffing-out-cancer/.

42. Veselkov, K.A., et al., (2014) Chemo-informatic strategy for imaging mass spectrometry based hyper-spectral profiling of lipid signatures in colorectal cancer. *Proceedings of the National Academy of Sciences*. DOI: 10.1073/pnas. 1310524111.

Chapter Sixteen - How Can We Win the War on Cancer?

1. Bayer, R., et al. (2013) Confronting the Sorry State of U.S. Health. *Science*. 341: 962-963.

2. American Society of Clinical Oncology (2014) *The State of Cancer Care in America: 2014*. Alexandria, VA: American Society of Clinical Oncology.

3. op cit. Bayer.

4. Kaiser, Jocelyn (2013) Varmus's Second Act. *Science*. 342: 416-419.

5. http://www.charitynavigator.org/index.cfm?bay=content.view&cpid=497.

6. Patel, Jyoti D., et al. (2014) Clinical Cancer Advances 2013: Annual Report on Progress against Cancer from the American Society of Clinical Oncology. *Journal of Clinical Oncology.* 32 (2) 129-160.

7. Emanuel, Ezekiel (2014) *Reinventing American Health Care: How the Affordable Care Act Will Improve Our Terribly Complex, Blatantly Unjust, Outrageously Expensive, Grossly Inefficient, Error Prone System.* New York: Public Affairs.

8. Lichtenstein, P., et al. (2000) Environmental and Heritable Factors in the Causation of Cancer—Analyses of Cohorts of Twins from Sweden, Denmark, and Finland. New *England Journal of Medicine.* 343 (2): 78-85.

9. Travado, Luzia, et al. (2012) Psycho-oncology and Advocacy in Cancer Care: An International Perspective. In Grassi, Luigi & Riba, Michelle. *Clinical Psycho-oncology: An International Perspective.* New York: Wiley-Blackwell.

INDEX

CPSIA information can be obtained at www.ICGtesting.com
Printed in the USA
LVOW08s1048190616

493237LV00002B/430/P